HAIR
marie claire

JOSETTE MILGRAM
TRANSLATED BY KIM ALLEN GLEED

HAIR
marie claire

HEARST BOOKS
A division of Sterling Publishing Co., Inc.

New York / London
www.sterlingpublishing.com

Contents

WE *ALL* HAVE THE RIGHT TO *BEAUTIFUL* HAIR!

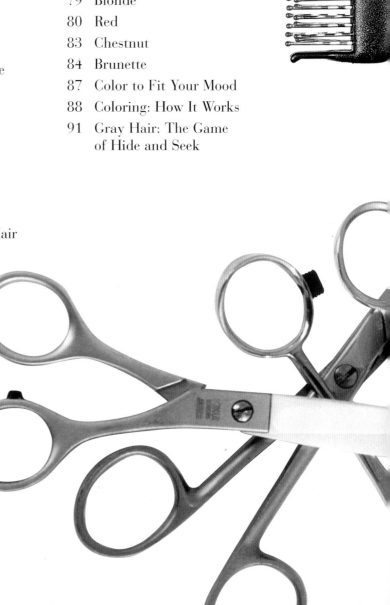

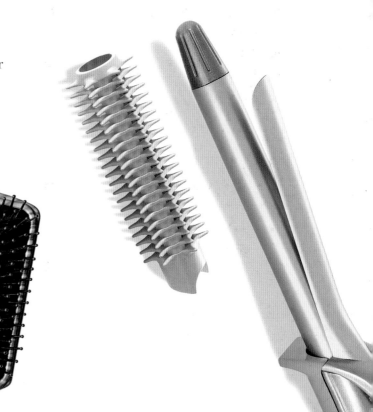

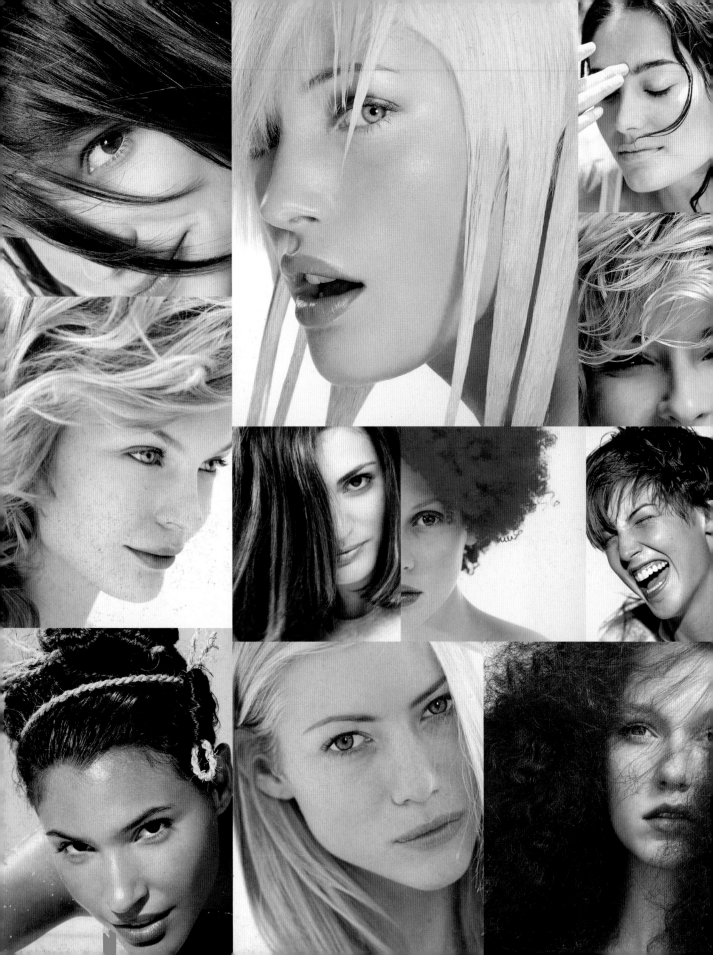

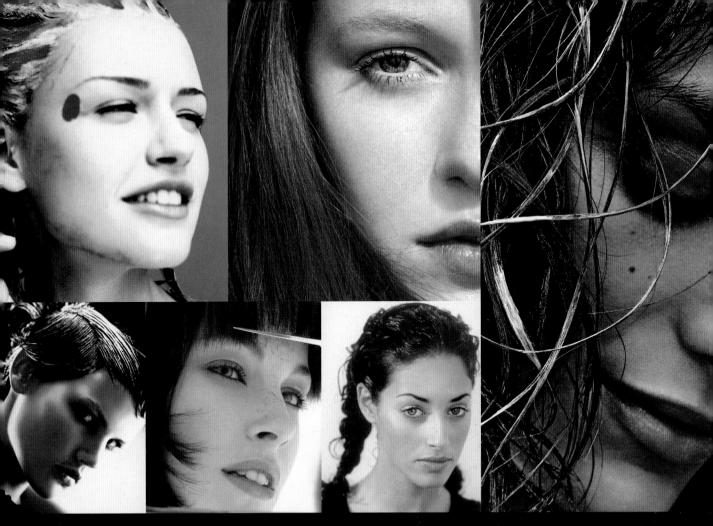

We *all* have the right to *beautiful* hair!

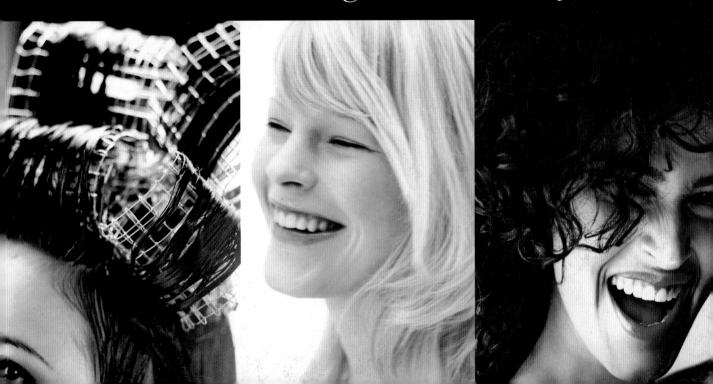

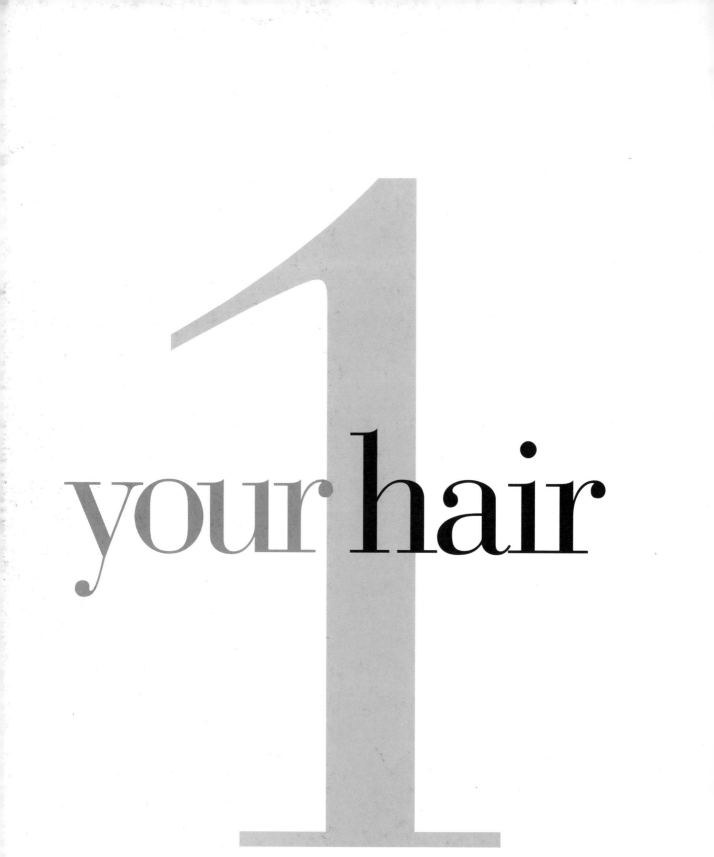

1 your hair

YOUR CROWNING GLORY

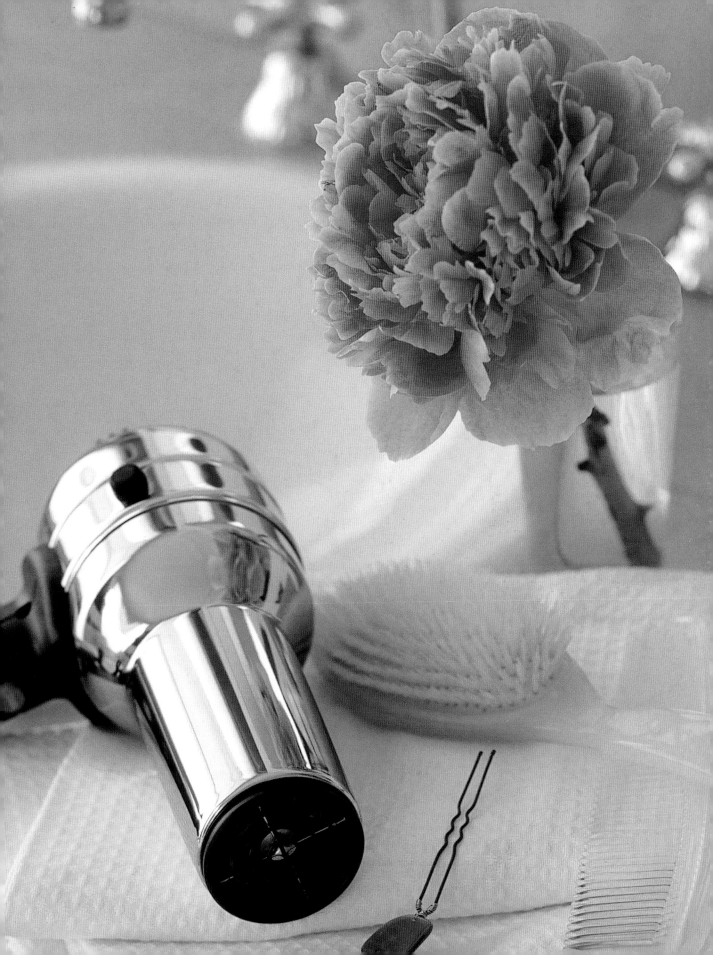

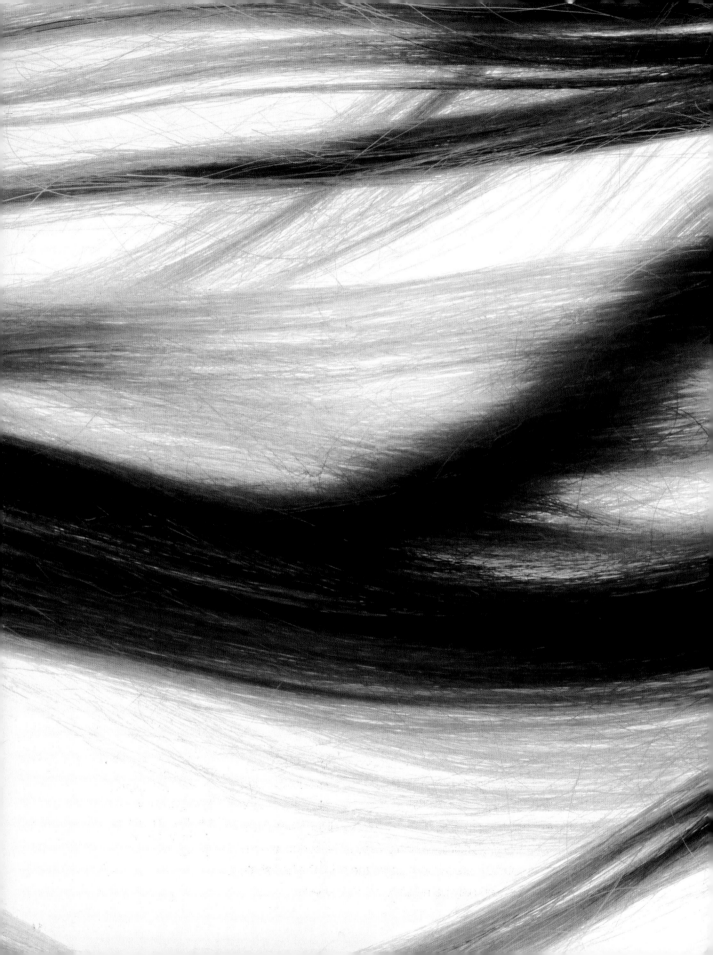

The secret life of hair

It often seems that our hair does exactly as it pleases. And here's why: From the hairline to the color, from texture to volume, everything is genetically programmed before birth.

IT'S AT THE ROOT, under the skin, where we find the **hair follicle,** the living part where hair is created.

It is a **biochemical factory** in every respect where intense activity is carried out: cells multiply faster there than anywhere else in the body and have an astonishing capacity for renewal.

THE SHAFT, the visible part of hair, is actually already dead. Each strand of hair has its own genetically programmed life cycle: a growing phase (called the anagen phase), which can last from a few months to seven years; a regression phase (called the cathagen phase) of a few weeks; and finally a resting phase (called the telogen phase) of three to four months, after which the hair falls out and the cycle begins again. The differences in life expectancy explain why some strands never seem to come in and others seem to stay forever. Thankfully, since we lose on average 20 to 80 per day (20,000 per year), our 100,000 to 150,000 hair follicles act perfectly independently of each other, with each root disposing of its own hair and then growing it again.

AN EXCEPTIONALLY STRONG MATERIAL: A tuft of 2,000 strands of healthy hair could easily lift over 65 pounds. This is thanks to keratin, a protein that winds extremely resistant fibers into a construction of overlapping scales, like tiles. Melanin is what gives hair its color, and the lipids bind it all together, forming the outer layer, or cuticle, which protects the cortex and the core. One important precaution: unlike the skin, the hair shaft, once damaged, can only be repaired on the surface.

Did you know?

- Certain lipids, called ceramides, are present in hair to help keep it healthy. Today we know how to recreate them identically thanks to cloning and add them to strengthening products.
- The average diameter of a strand of hair is 0.002 inch.
- At 8 inches long, laid flat, the hair on your head could cover a surface of nearly 20 square feet.
- Hair is elastic: It lengthens up to 50 percent when wet.
- Hair is hydrophilic: It lengthens or shortens based on the humidity in the air.

What your hair says about you

An extremely knowledgeable informant, each strand of our hair tells our genetic history, as well as our emotional one, every day. Here are some of the secrets your hair keeps.

ONE SINGLE STRAND of hair reveals our complete identity, including a genetic map. The root, irrigated with blood vessels, is teeming with the most in-depth information about our DNA as well as our mood.

First and foremost, DNA has an incredible longevity, and it keeps everything in its memory for centuries. All you need is one strand of hair to discover crucial information on how Beethoven and Napoleon died or what color hair Ramses II had (it was strawberry blonde, enhanced by henna).

STRESS shows over time. Since hair grows approximately 0.01 inch per day, all you need to do is locate a small weakened area along the shaft to precisely identify the time you were worried. The hair bulb registers the most miniscule variation in our diet and lifestyle: on about two-and-a-half inches of hair, you can trace what you consumed over the past six months.

MALE OR FEMALE, they display their color: Yes, hair has a sex. The percentage of testosterone in men's hair gives the secret away instantly.

ADVICE FROM A DERMATOLOGIST

Here's what you see at the root:
- Sebaceous glands (sebum lubricates the hair fiber and makes it shiny and supple)
- The erector pili muscle (which causes the hair on your head to stand on end if you are cold or afraid)
- The papilla, connected to the nervous system (where reactions to stress come from)

Hair—another victim of tobacco

Spending time in a smoky atmosphere doesn't just make our hair smell bad (no other odor holds tighter to the fibers of hair). The free radicals contained in cigarette smoke weaken hair, which is very sensitive to this type of pollution.

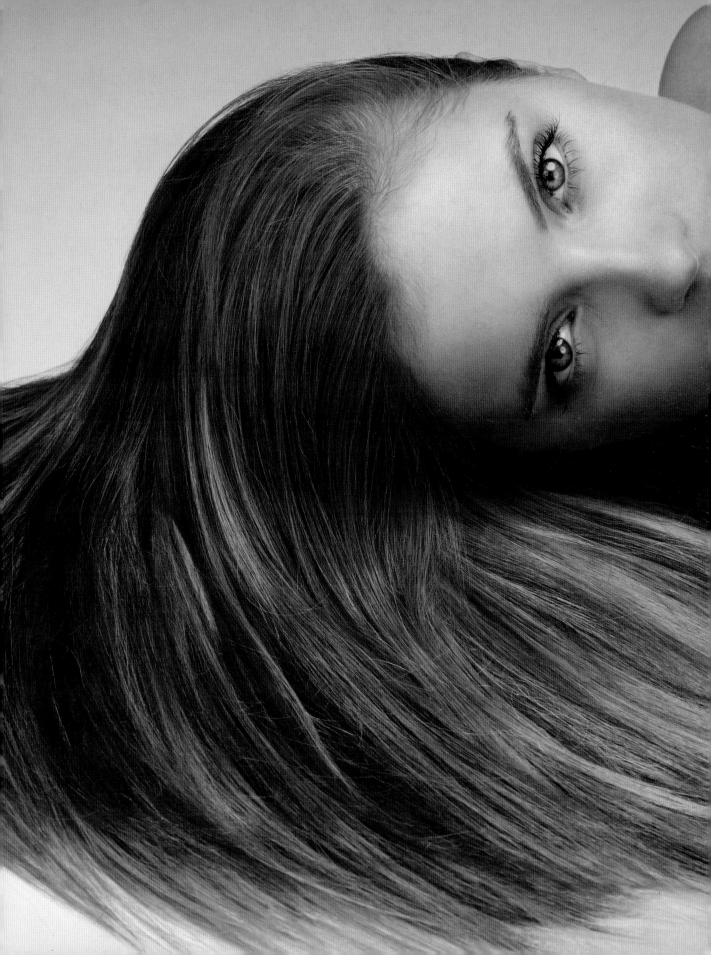

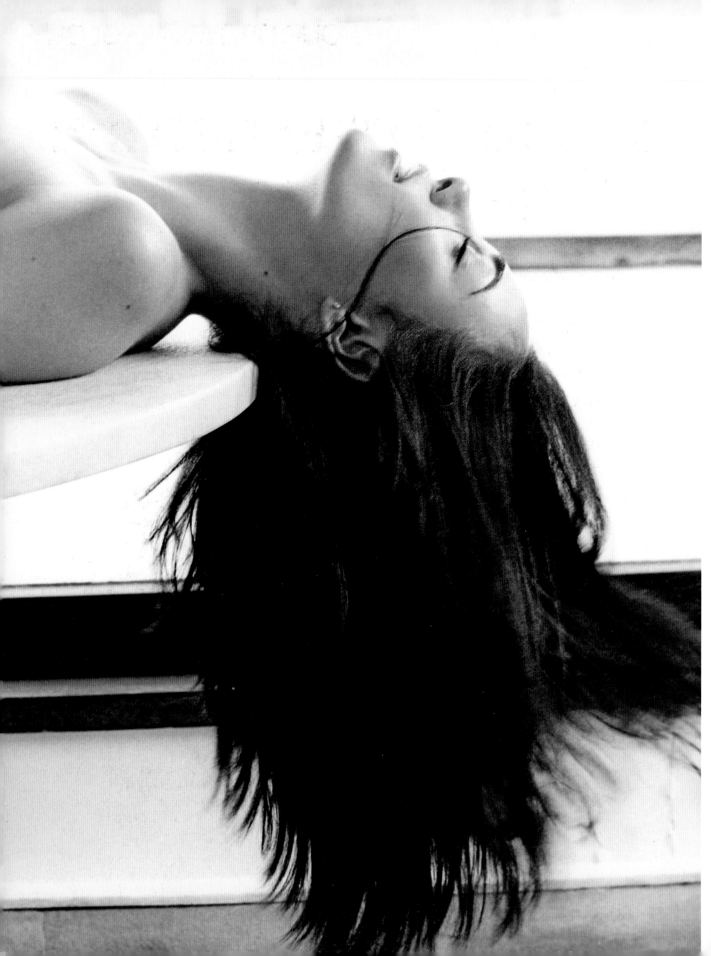

Your hair's true nature: A quick diagnosis

Hair is genetically programmed, but strongly influenced by our lifestyle and the stresses of our environment. Truly understanding the nature of hair is the best way for you to make the most of it.

NORMAL Normal hair is naturally healthy and shiny and stays clean longer. But pollution and variations in our hormonal cycles can cause temporary changes to hair.

DRY Fragile and dull, dry hair suffers from a marked lack of sebum, which is what smooths the scales on the shaft and gives hair its sleek look. This is particularly common in curly hair, whose irregular surface makes even distribution of the natural lubricant difficult.

OILY Sebum is wonderful . . . unless you have too much. Perspiration, stress, overproduction of testosterone, and certain medications are just some of the triggers. The scalp is actually the part of the body with the most sebaceous glands, and they're ready to make themselves known at any moment: All you have to do is touch your hair a bit too frequently. Keep brushing and massaging to a minimum.

COMBINATION Oily at the roots, dry at the ends: Combination hair is a true hassle and is mainly the result of poorly selected treatments. Most of the time, combination hair is naturally oily hair that has been damaged at the ends by repeated coloring or perming. On the other hand, if naturally dry hair is shampooed too aggressively and the scalp becomes stripped, the seborrhea is stimulated and roots become oily.

ADVICE FROM A RESEARCHER
We are not good at evaluating ourselves: Most of us imagine we have thin hair even though, objectively, it is not the case.

The nature of our hair changes on average every six years
Therefore, we must adapt our hair-care regimens accordingly. Life in general and diet in particular play a key role: For example, the more fats we eat, the oilier our hair will be.

The world of color

The number one beauty ace up your sleeve, the absolute weapon of femininity, your hair is a full-fledged fashion accessory that seduces in every hue. Here, we explore color.

Where does color come from? Color is derived from a skillful mixture of two types of melanin, namely **eumelanin** and **pheomelanin.** These seeds are carefully sown in incredible color laboratories called **melanocytes,** situated at the heart of the capillary bulb, and are all that it takes to create the entire spectrum of colors, from platinum to raven. The genetically programmed color code is then transmitted to the **keratinocytes,** the cells that make the hair.

MELANIN MAKES THE DIFFERENCE. The chemistry that has given birth to the myriad shades of hair remains a mystery: Why are Asian black and Scandinavian blonde made up of the same melanin (eumelanin, the darkest, which varies from brownish-red to black), while shades of red are composed of pheomelanin (the lightest, with a yellow-red tint), which is also found in blondes? The answer is in the infinite complexity of the combinations of genetic markers.

BLONDE The color of movie stars and the symbol of certain types of femininity (from the angelic innocent to the *femme fatale* vamp), blonde has a unique way of capturing the light.

RED From the same family as blonde, with shades of copper and orange, this is a feisty palette with an intriguing range of tones.

CHESTNUT Dark blonde or light brown (colorists don't necessarily use the same words as we do).

BRUNETTE The absolute shiniest shade, full of deep seduction and the mystery of nocturnal reflections.

GRAY Technically, gray hair does not exist—it's actually an optical illusion created by our original color and our first white strands.

WHITE This is the effect of zero pigment after, for no clear reason, the production of melanin stops. And it can happen just as easily before thirty as after sixty!

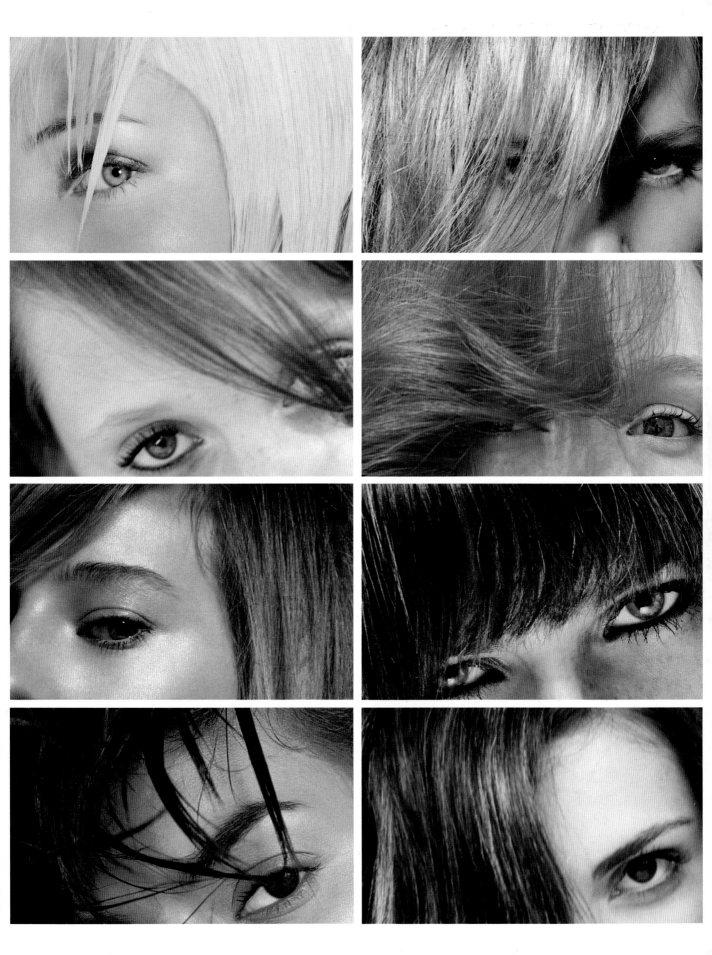

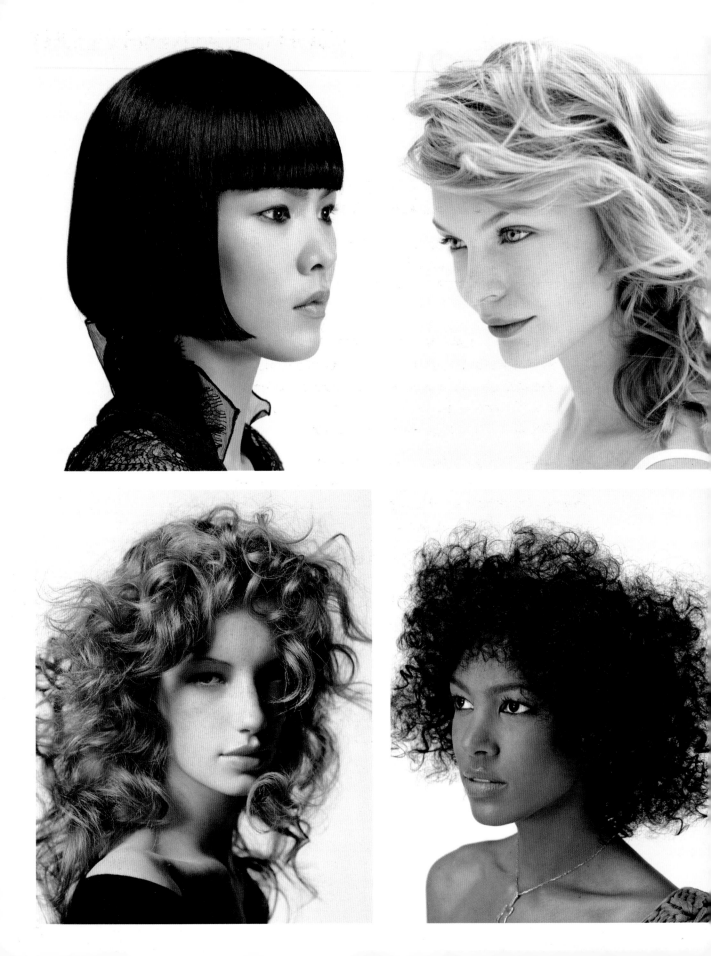

All the textures

Fine and sleek, rebellious or luxuriant—your hair's texture also reveals your well-established genetic codes. Understand your hair's texture to make the most of it.

THE FLATTER A HAIR IS, THE MORE IT WILL CURL!
The shape of the capillary shaft, the "mold" formed at the root under the scalp, is what determines hair texture. If you look at it under a microscope, it is oval-shaped and more or less flat depending on the type of growth and implantation.

STRAIGHT A round capillary shaft is characteristic of straight hair. The more symmetrical it is, the closer it is to Asian hair, the paragon of straightness and the type with the largest diameter. European hair also has this type of structure.

WAVY AND CURLY The capillary shaft of wavy and curly hair is less round and more flat, with all variations of an oval coexisting even on the same head. Certain areas on the scalp may produce hair that is curlier than others.

COARSE AND CURLY The capillary shaft is flattest in African hair, which is characterized by extremely tight curls. To demonstrate this phenomenon, think about what happens when you flatten a ribbon against the blade of a pair of scissors to curl it when you're wrapping a present.

Each has its own rhythm!
The world record for speed of growth is held by Asian hair: over half an inch per month, but with a weak density. It grows straight, perpendicular to the head. European hair grows slightly less than half an inch per month, but it is much thicker. African hair, which only grows about a third of an inch per month, progresses as tendrils parallel to the scalp.

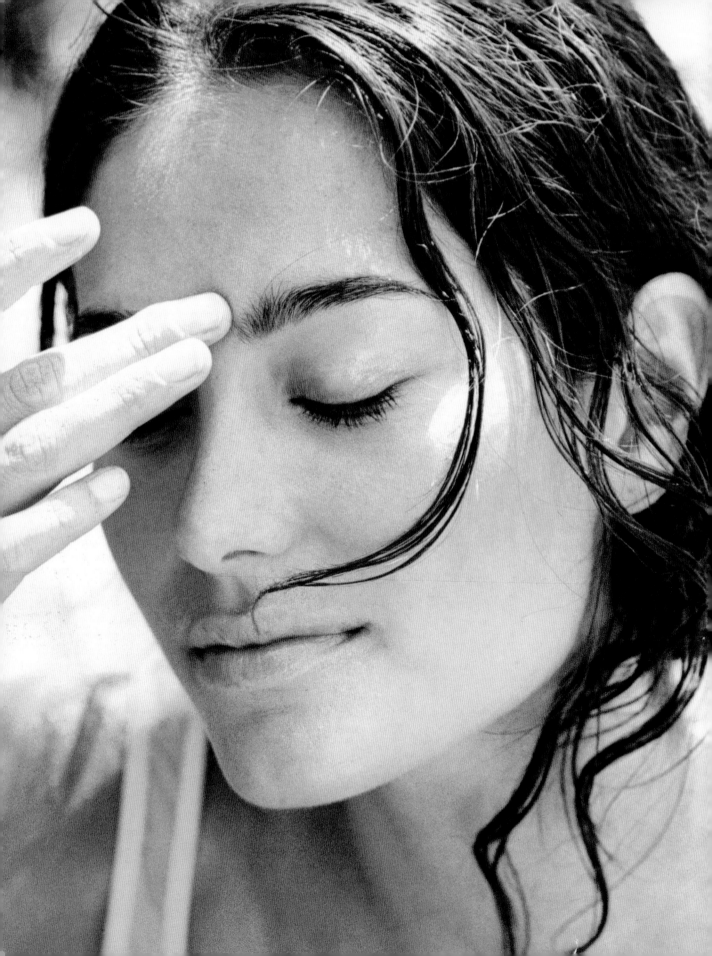

Beauty at 20 . . . and at every age

An absolutely faithful reflection of all the stages of womanhood, the state of our hair does not have to give away our age. Thankfully, anti-aging treatments can work wonders on hair.

HORMONES PLAY A ROLE Estrogen is a key player: Its presence at the root, via hormonal receptors, makes women's hair grow faster than men's. From the onset of puberty to the use of birth control pills, everything that interferes with our hormonal balance has consequences on the state of our hair.

ADOLESCENCE The influx of testosterone is responsible for seborrhea—and oily hair—which causes headaches for many teenage girls—and sometimes even limited hair loss.

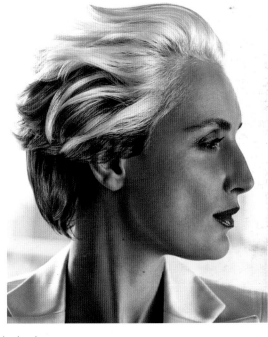

BEFORE (AND AFTER) BABY The luscious hair of mothers-to-be is due to the abundance of female hormones (estrogen), which slow down the life cycle of hair. New hairs arrive and old ones remain, resulting in a blissful time for hair and skin as well. Once the baby is born, however, the hormones relax their vigilance and, as a result, hair falls out, sometimes in large quantities, after childbirth. Thankfully, the situation stabilizes within a few weeks.

MENOPAUSE As a result of reduced female hormones, hair risks falling out. As long as they are mixed in the correct proportions, substitutive treatments which keeps testosterone in check curb this phenomenon. And new anti-aging treatments are great at adding body and texture to hair.

ADVICE FROM A DERMATOLOGIST
In certain cases, you can get a prescription hormone treatment gel that is applied directly to the roots of the hair.

The future of hair

The solutions of tomorrow are being prepared today in secret laboratories. Jean-Michel Sturla, director of scientific coordination at the L'Oréal Hair Research Laboratory, highlights the leads that could transform our dreams into reality.

AN ABSOLUTE MASTERY OF FORM, the most beautiful sleek reflection, hair that's soft to touch, that remains supple, that looks vibrant, and above all, has endless shine?

It's on the way! You have naturally dull hair? You can have "naturally" shiny. Naturally dry hair? You can have "naturally" soft. Naturally lifeless hair? We're going to give you "natural" volume. Rebellious hair? Well-styled curls!

We are moving closer and closer to **undetectable solutions that yield maximum results.** The star here is not the product but the results it provides. And for that, research is mobilized on every front. Women are becoming experts—and more demanding about product performance; expectations have never been higher.

It's not about pure functionality anymore; instead, researchers are emphasizing high-quality, gourmet ingredients.

Hair is going to be treated as a subject, as if it has a personality, with an attention that goes beyond aesthetics. Hair must be beautiful, of course, but it also has to smell good, be nice to touch. **It must appeal to all the senses.**

ADVICE FROM PATRICIA PINEAU, L'ORÉAL RESEARCHER

- **HAVE YOUR NATURAL COLOR AGAIN?**
Yes, if biological recoloration becomes possible by reawakening "sleeping" melanocytes.

- **CHANGE THE TEXTURE?**
Possible, thanks to progress in genetics and epigenesis, a modulation in genes by environmental factors such as nutrition. Extensive studies have shown that diet influences the health of hair, and that nutritional supplements have a cosmetic benefit.

- **WHAT ABOUT PERFUMES?**
Ancient civilizations perfumed and nourished their hair with ointments—a lead which still requires further research.

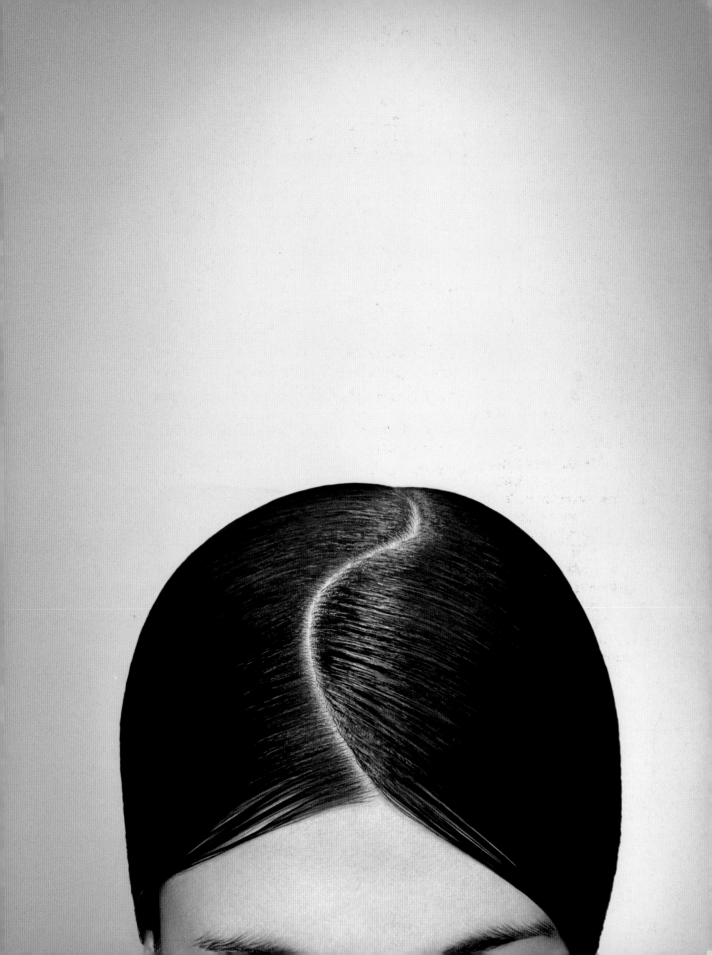

2

hair care

FAVORITE TREATMENTS

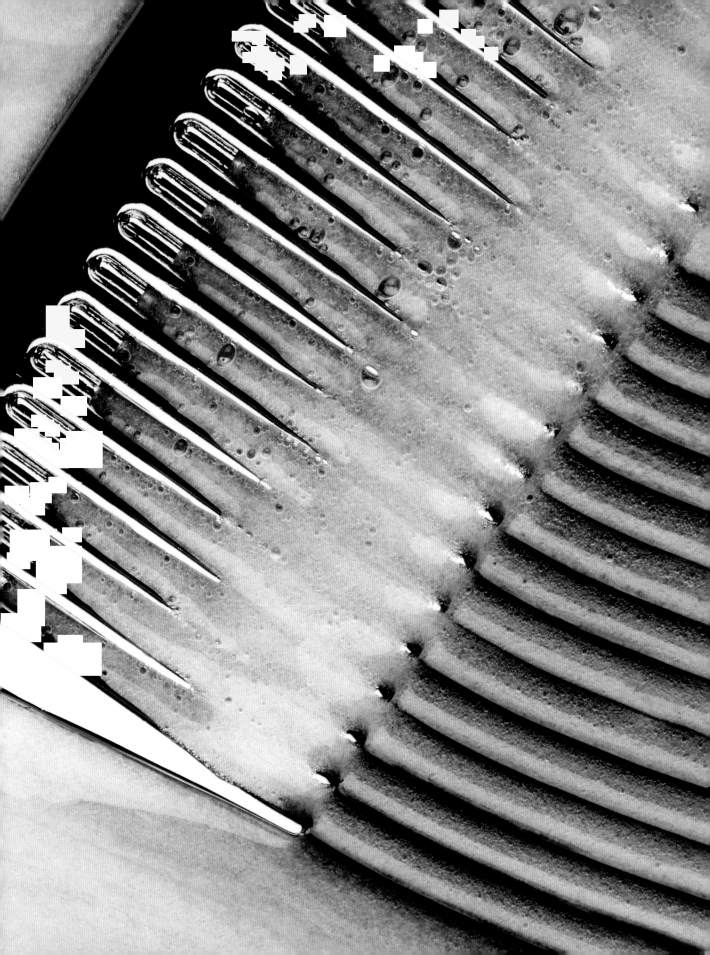

Treat your hair right every day and respect its true nature.

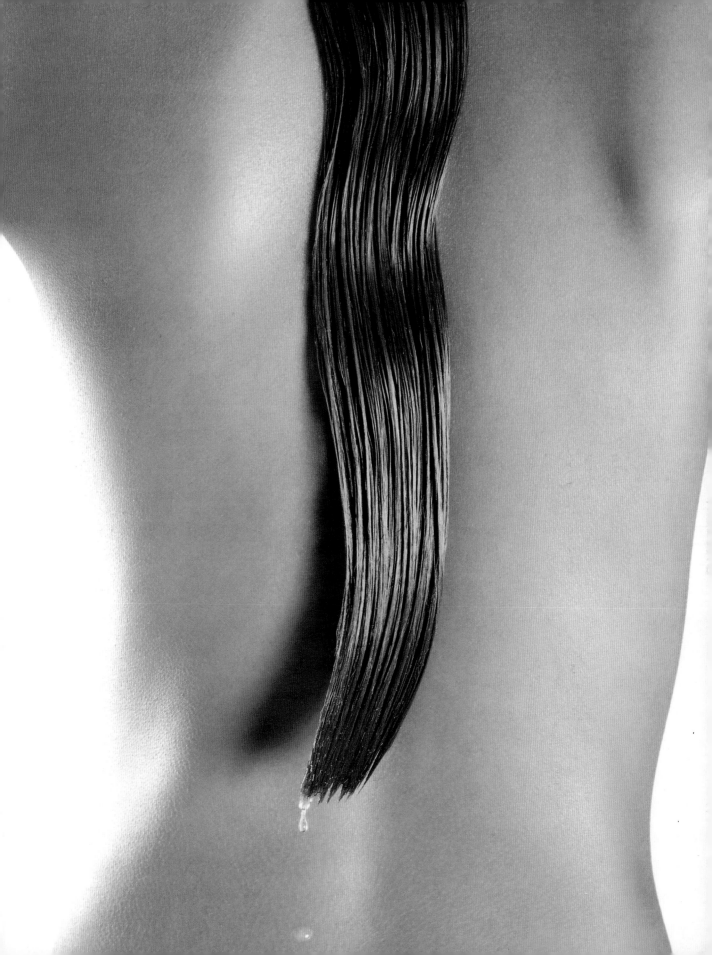

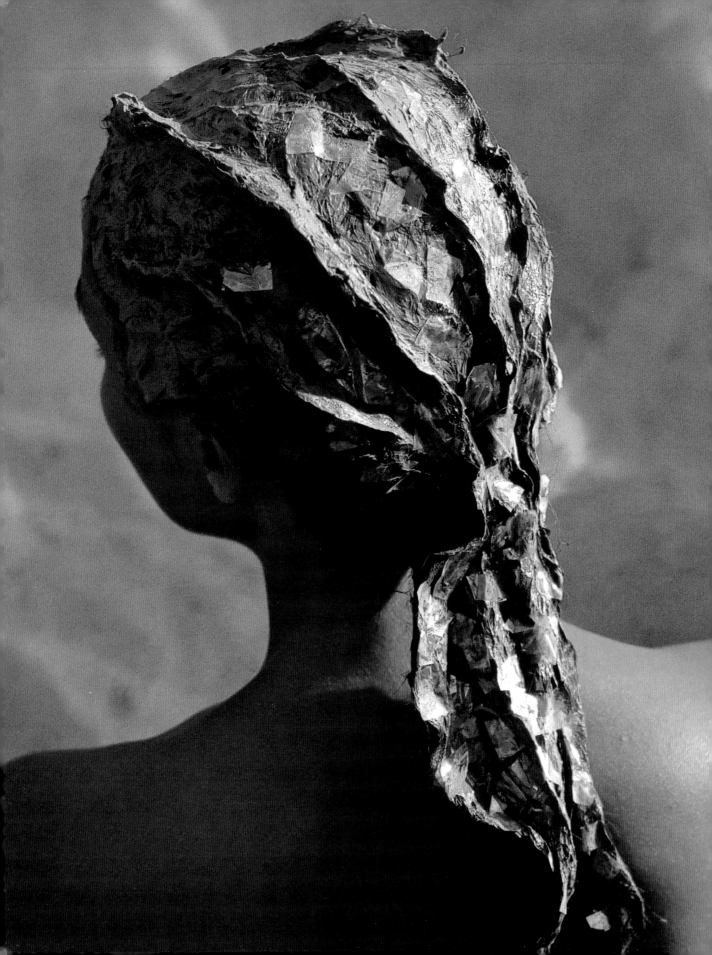

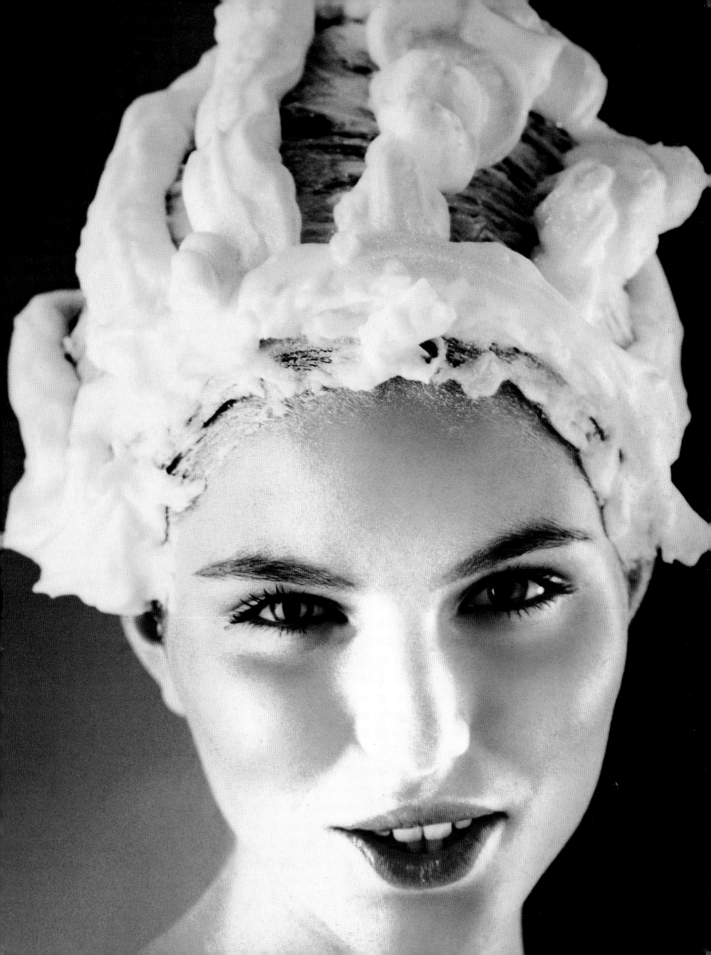

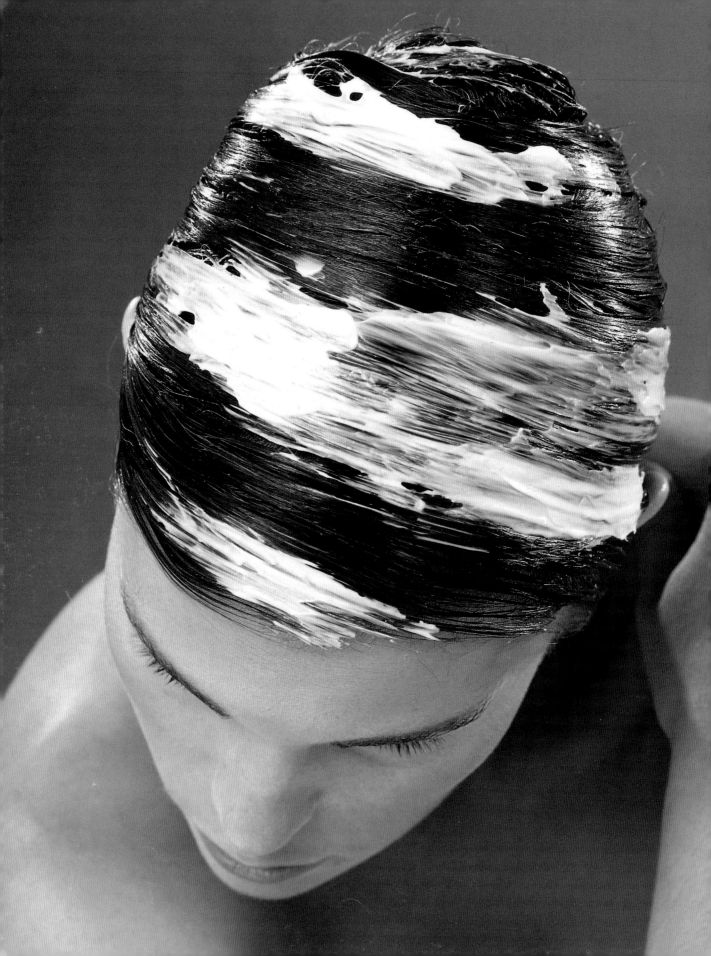

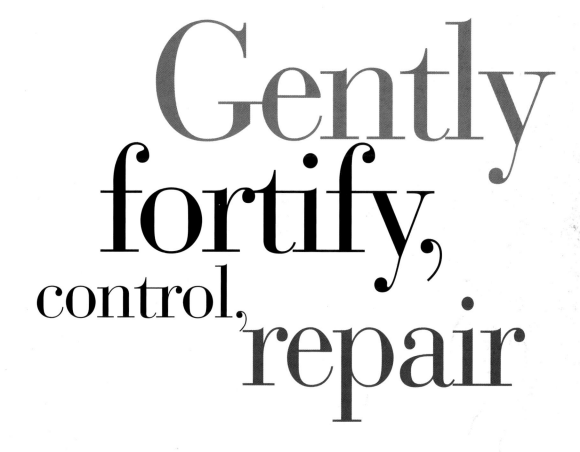

Gently fortify, control, repair

Nice and clean

From selecting a good shampoo to deciding how often to use it and how long to rinse based on the quality of your water, most day-to-day beauty tasks are far from trivial.

ADVICE FROM A DERMATOLOGIST
Pollution has a negative effect on hair health: The scalp becomes sensitized to it and as a result, requires more frequent shampooing especially if you are exposed to a great deal of it. But you should only use gentle, high-quality products that respect the natural bacterial flora of the scalp.

Water help!
Hard water is tough on hair. If it is not possible to install a water-softening filter where you live, a vinegar rinse (one capful in two cups of tap water) will wash away any traces of sediment.

CHOOSE A GOOD SHAMPOO Pick a shampoo based on the **condition of your scalp** (sensitive, dry, oily), since the ends of your hair can be treated after shampooing. You can alternate with a more specialized shampoo for volume or shine.

The newest generation of two-in-one shampoos, made using surfactants, ceramides, silicones and polymers, combine detangling, softening, smoothing, and refreshing. But avoid using them too frequently, or you will overdose the roots.

Dry hair is thirsty for very gentle products (but avoid extra-conditioning products formulated for babies, as little ones do not have any sebum). In the case of **oily hair**, which gets dirty quickly, stay away from harsh products, which can cause a "rebound" effect: overproduction of sebum in the scalp that then works its way down the strand and weighs hair down. The scalp must be nourished and hydrated rather than attacked. Gentle formulas for oily roots are best for **combination hair**, while special formulas for color-treated hair bring cohesion back to the shaft's scales and extend the life of your color. Finally, **anti-dandruff shampoos**, alternated with more gentle formulas, provide excellent results.

HOW OFTEN? Many of us feel compelled to shampoo daily, but every other day (or even every two days) should suffice. Of course, washing too infrequently risks suffocating the scalp with an accumulation of oil, which slows growth, encourages dandruff, and can even lead to hair loss.

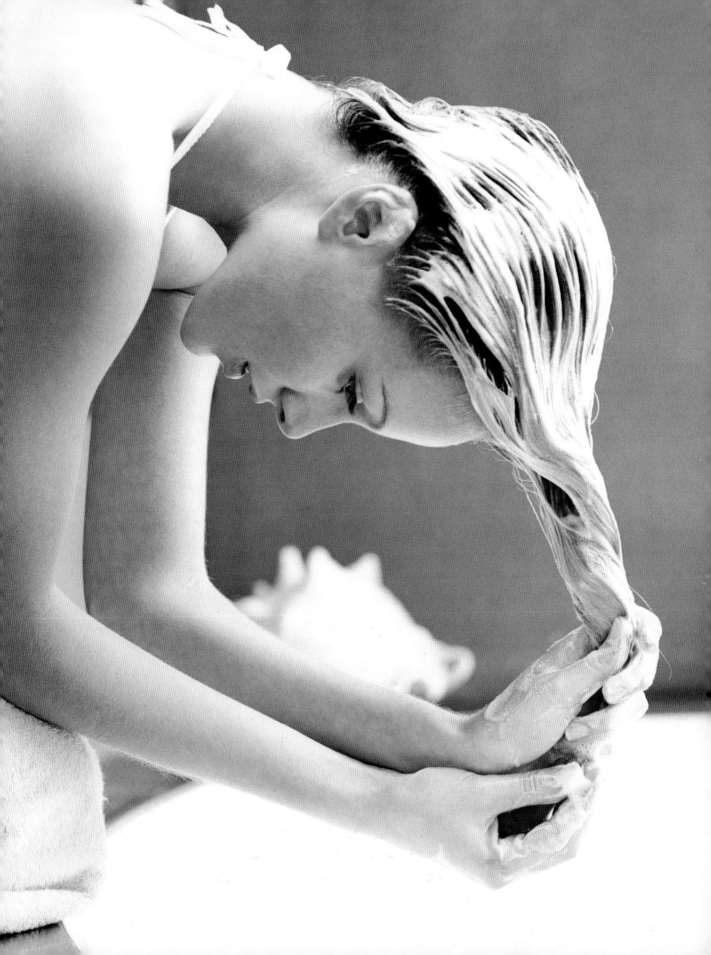

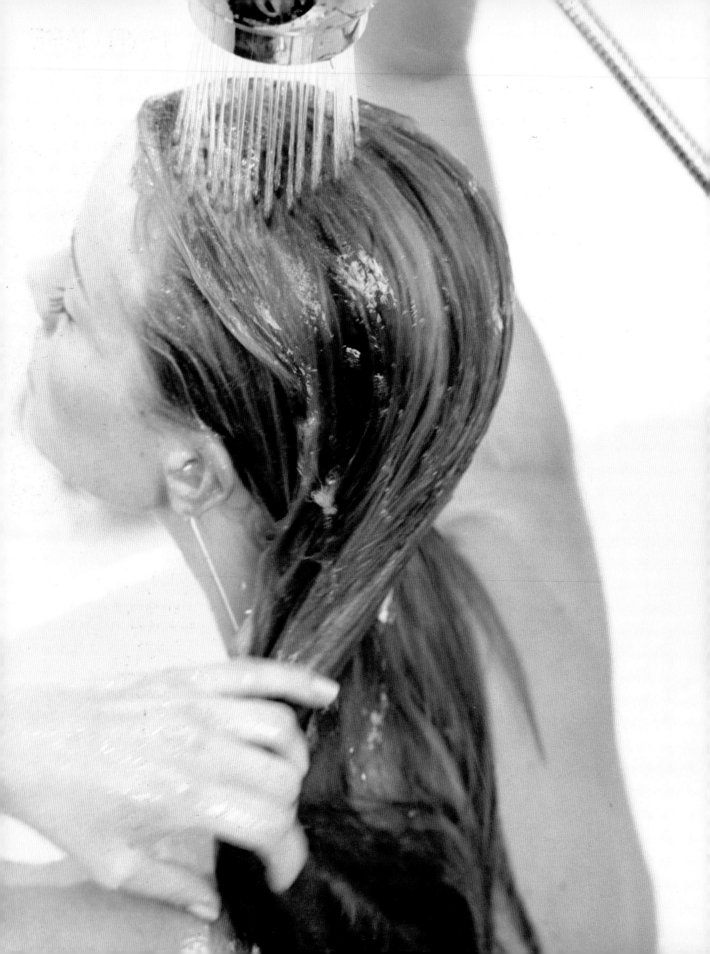

EIGHT EASY STEPS TO SQUEAKY-CLEAN HAIR

1 BRUSH YOUR HAIR before washing to help the water penetrate and to eliminate some of the impurities and product residue.

2 THOROUGHLY WET YOUR HAIR. Your entire head must be evenly saturated.

3 BE CAREFUL how much shampoo you use. It's not the quantity that counts; in fact, too much shampoo can weaken hair. Start with a grape-size amount and work from the scalp to the ends of the hair, adding water as needed, but without bringing the ends back up to the scalp (this can cause tangling, and your hair won't get as clean).

4 MASSAGE the scalp with your fingertips (but don't scrub—it weakens the roots) to evenly distribute the shampoo and stimulate circulation.

5 ONE WASH OR TWO? There is no one-size-fits-all rule on this. If you wash often, one shampoo is sufficient. One exception, however, is oily hair (because sebum prevents lather on the first application, it's best to repeat). And if hair is exposed to pollution, the first wash rinses away impurities while the second focuses on treating the problem (dandruff, seborrhea, etc.).

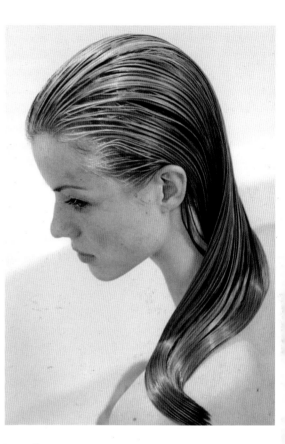

6 LATHER is a simple signal that your shampoo is working effectively. Today's shampoos are no longer abrasive; they don't lift the scales on the hair shaft, weakening it and making it more porous and static prone.

7 RINSE THOROUGHLY with your head back under the shower, just like at the salon, focusing on the roots. That is the only way of removing all traces of shampoo so that your hair remains cleaner longer. In addition, it allows you to remove dead skin cells on the scalp, which are often mistaken for dandruff.

8 A SPLASH OF COLD WATER après shampoo is a must for extra shine—not an old wives' tale. It smooths out the scales on the hair.

ADVICE FROM STYLIST ÉRIC PFALZGRAF
It is best to shampoo in two steps (two small shampoos instead of one large), first using a general shampoo, and then one designed to treat a specific need. If you can bear it, use the Scottish shower method, switching from hot water, to warm, and then to cold.

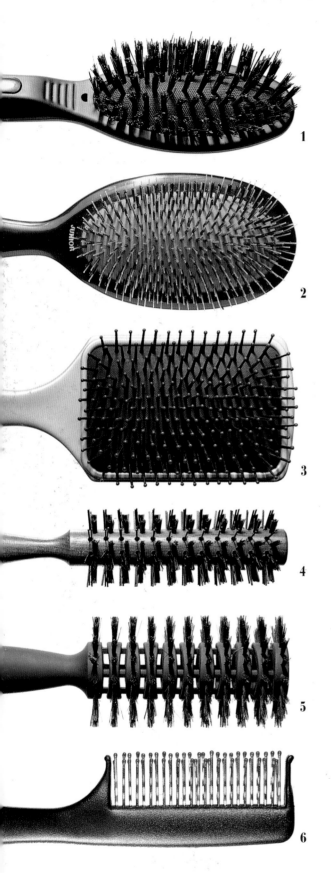

The must-have tools

Brushes and combs, irons and dryers—professional tools for a true beauty strategy.

1 All brushes with natural hair bristles, like this very practical **boar's hair** model, help prevent static electricity.

2 Mason-Pearson, the Rolls-Royce of brushes, is the great **English classic** that blends nylon and boar bristles on a rubber-cushion.

3 The **paddle of top stylists:** This completely synthetic brush is especially good for long and medium-length hair.

4 Perfect for **short hair,** this one blends short natural and synthetic bristles for professional results when blowdrying.

5 This brush's **anti-static** treated boar bristles and open cylinder are excellent for dispersing heat while blowdrying.

6 **Steel teeth** for better combing: unbeatable for parting hair and distributing treatments and styling products from roots to ends.

. . . And for all of them, good hygiene! A weekly bath in diluted gentle shampoo washes your combs and brushes and rids them of impurities.

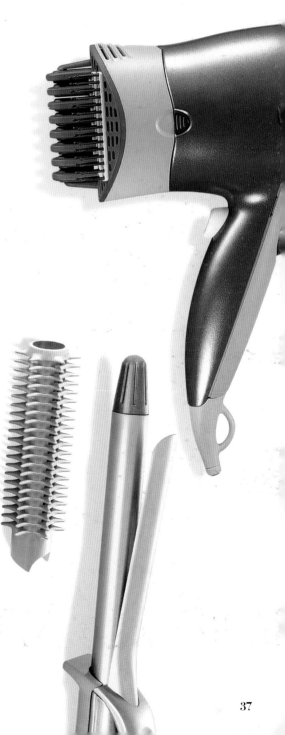

A smoothing iron (above) or curling iron (below) are today's absolute beauty must-haves. They are the perfect complements to exceptional styling products.

BRUSHING TIPS Brush in the **morning** to tidy up your hair after sleeping on it all night, and again at **night** to eliminate styling products and accumulated dust.

The myth of **100 strokes** when brushing should be kicked to the curb: Overbrushing stimulates sebum production and can also cause split ends.

COMBS 101 Choose natural materials, such as horn, rather than synthetic ones, which have a tendency to cause static electricity.

DRY WITHOUT DRYING OUT Drying your hair with your dryer on the **cool** setting prevents thermal shock while still boosting volume, which is difficult to obtain by **air-drying**.

EXTREME VARIATIONS IN TEMPERATURE pose a real threat to our hair. A dryer on a setting that's too hot (100 degrees is already dangerous) can singe the hair and cause grave damage by breaking the scales.

CURLING IRONS and **SMOOTHING IRONS** (indispensable for sleek styles) must only be used on hair that is completely dry to avoid thermal damage.

A HEAT SHIELD for your dryer is also a must-have. Styling with the control of a **nozzle or diffuser** guarantees a safe **blowdry**.

After you shampoo: What your hair craves

Our hair is greedy. Taking a minute or two before drying can correct the negative effects of hard water and give your hair all the shine it deserves!

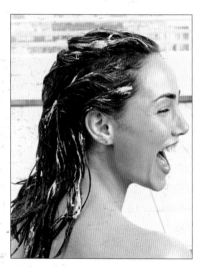

TREATMENTS FOR YOUR HAIR

Conditioners are a true gift to your hair. They nourish the ends and provide brilliant shine. Conditioners are composed of special agents that should not be used at the roots—shampoo has already done its work here, and conditioner will only weigh it down.

There are many different formulas and textures, and you should choose a conditioner based on your current needs as well as the weather and season in which you'll be using it.

Lotions and **sprays** work to **detangle** hair by acting on the electrostatic properties inside the hair shaft. Charged with the same electric charge, strands of hair will repel each other.

A **deep-conditioning mask** provides a total cocoon. Hair is pampered and so are you, as long as you have a bit of time to spare.

Conditioning is as close to hair nutrition as you can get. It should not be too light in texture—if it is, you'll have the impression that it is not doing anything—but it is also important not to weigh down your hair. So how long to leave conditioner in before rinsing? A minute should do the trick, but depending on cultural habits, it can range from a few minutes to as long as you please!

ADVICE FROM STYLIST JEAN-CLAUDE GALLON
What you do after you shampoo is very important. Even if you are in a hurry and you don't have enough time to let conditioner really absorb, you should still use it. It's better to rinse out conditioner quickly than to ignore it!

A secret . . .
A hot, wet towel (dampen it, then warm it in the microwave for a minute) will boost the positive effects of conditioner. Condition your hair and wrap the towel around your head for ten minutes before rinsing.

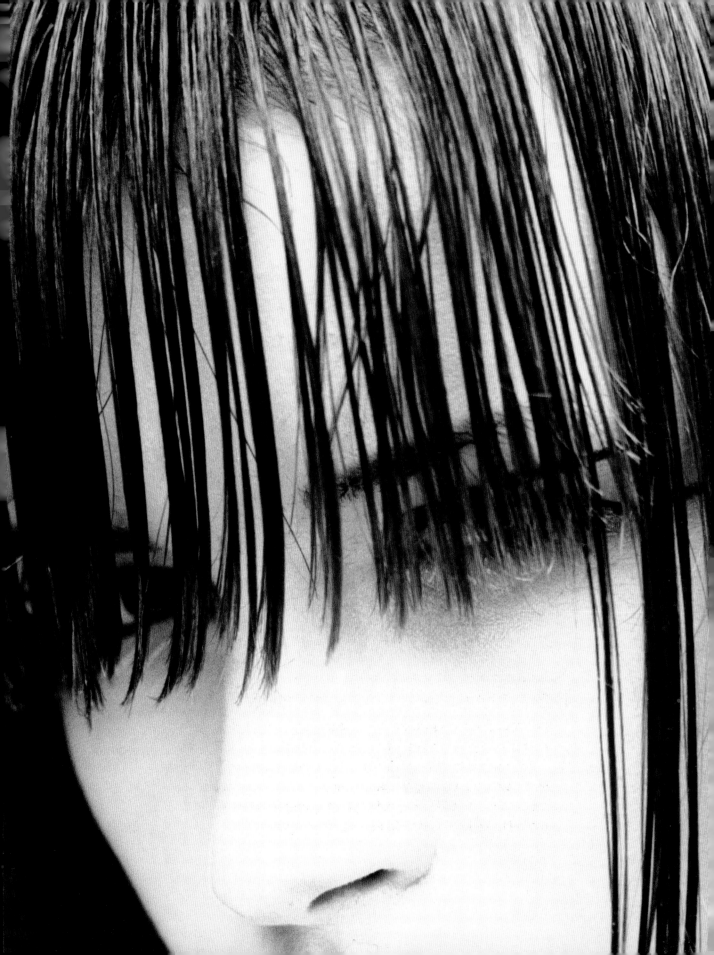

The perfect blowout

Want to smooth your out-of-control frizz?
Here's an easy three-step solution!

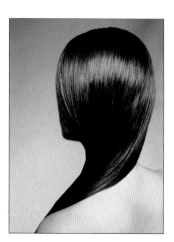

1 **TAMING** rebellious hair can be tricky. Begin by combing a leave-in smoothing product into wet hair, which will help you straighten hair while adding shine.

2 **TOWEL-DRY** to remove as much moisture as possible, then dry hair about 70 percent with a blow-dryer on a cool setting. You can use your fingers to continue to tame your hair, starting at the roots and moving to the ends. Add a few drops of smoothing serum (three to ten, depending on the length of your hair) before combing it again.

3 **USING A FLAT BRUSH**, moving from roots to ends, dry your hair. Place a section of hair on the brush with the bristles pointing out, and turn your dryer inwards toward the brush so the two are facing each other. Dry along the length of the hair as you brush down. The results are smooth and natural.

ADVICE FROM A STYLIST
To make sure that your sleek shine lasts even if the weather report predicts waves, use an anti-humidity hair spray before going outdoors, which keeps frizz at bay.

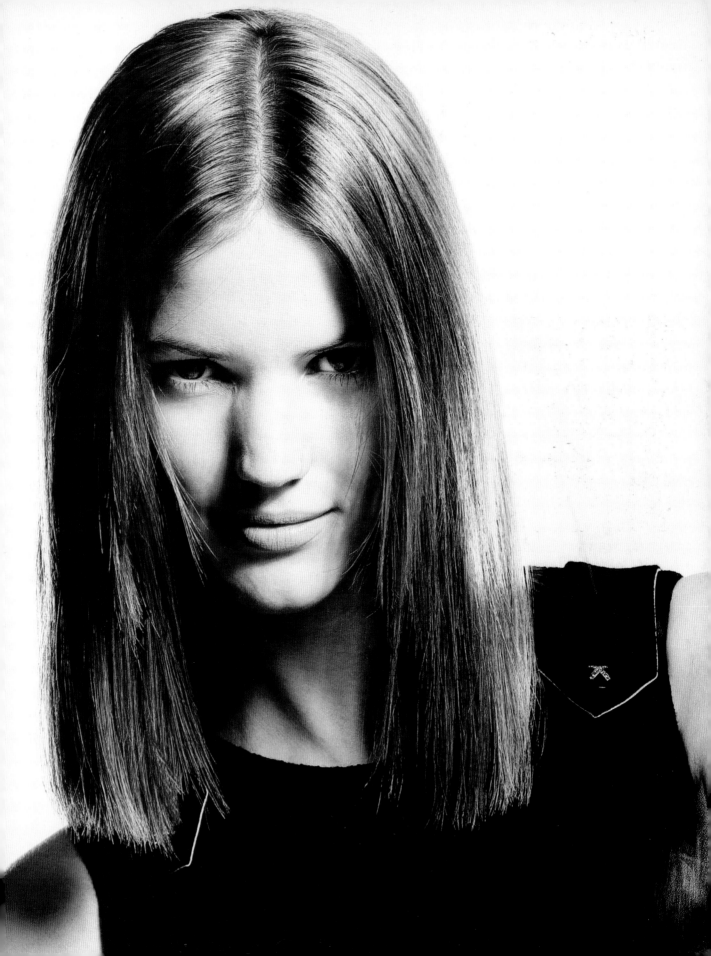

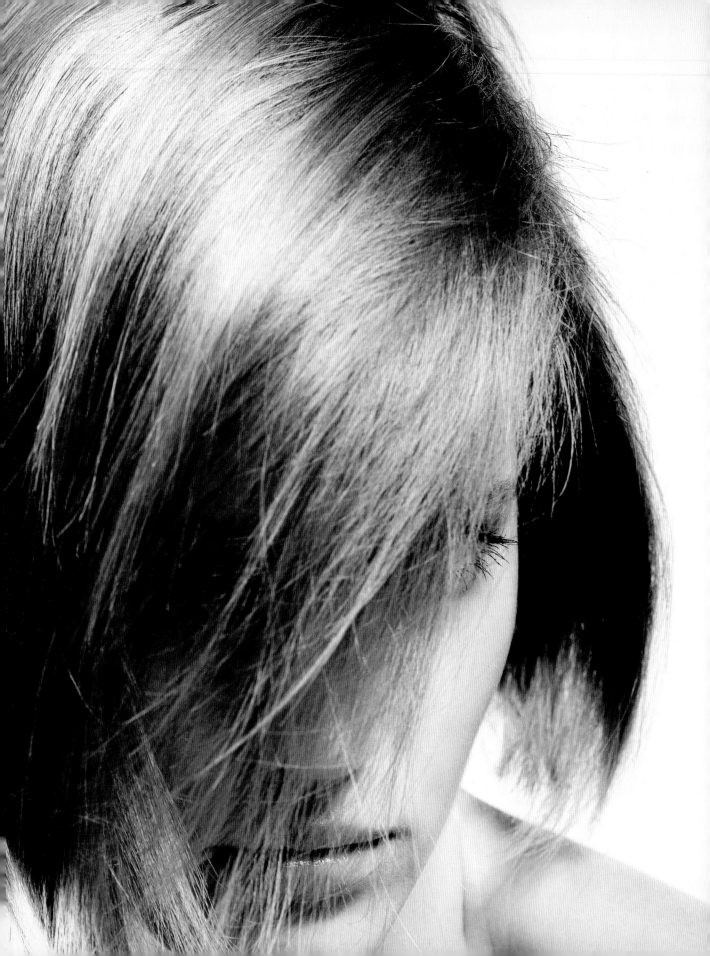

Boost volume with your blowdryer

Here's the magic recipe for everyone plagued by fine, limp, oily hair with only one wish: a bit of lift!

1 After detangling (which you've done only to the ends to avoid making the roots oily), apply **volumizing MOUSSE** using a comb, section by section, from the roots to the ends. Be careful not to use too much, though, because it will have exactly the opposite effect of the one you want.

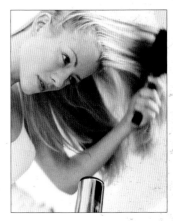

ADVICE FROM STYLIST JEAN-MARC MANAITIS Do not rub wet hair which, once tangled, will become impossible to style. Hair should be 70 percent dry before you use the blow-dryer. Let hair dry in an absorbent towel and pre-dry it to avoid the trauma of a too-hot dryer on soaking wet hair. Limit the amount of time you use the dryer, which, contrary to popular opinion, can reduce your hair's volume!

2 For a natural lift at the roots: **FLIP YOUR HEAD OVER,** drying first at the nape of your neck, which moves your hair in the opposite direction of how it naturally grows. Do this in three steps: first, with your head down, move the dryer from the base of your neck to the top of your head. Second, begin the same maneuver from right to left then left to right to force the hairs in the opposite direction at the root level and give them good volume. Finally, shake your head vigorously as you dry, sending the air from the dryer in every direction.

3 Spritz hair with a volumizing spray, then finish working with the dryer. **Hold large sections of hair away from your scalp** and dry the spray with the dryer.

Successful curls

Whatever your hair type, these tips will produce gorgeous results!

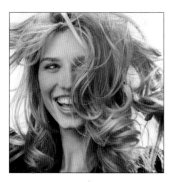

FOR NATURALLY CURLY OR PERMED HAIR, apply a styling treatment specifically designed to enhance curls and give your hair energy and elasticity. **Apply a mousse formulated to reinforce curls,** scrunching it in with your fingertips before distributing it with a comb. Then run your fingers through your hair to re-emphasize the shape of your curls.

Wipe the extra mousse off your hands and turn your **dryer, fitted with a diffuser, on the lowest setting.** Begin with your head flipped over, drying from top to bottom, root to tip, then flip your head back over, continuing to scrunch your hair and shape your curls with your fingers as you dry.

FOR STRAIGHT HAIR, there is only one option if you want curls: **a curling iron!** On hair that is still slightly damp, wind sections around your curling iron and then carefully comb out. The size of the curls will depend on the thickness of the hair you place in the curling iron. Twirl your hair around the iron and leave it there for one minute max. When your entire head is curled, allow curls to cool before spraying your hair with hairspray.

STYLIST'S TIP
If you prefer the effect of the mousse to be less pronounced, wait until hair is fully dry before applying the product. Use sparingly: soft hair is much sexier than stiff.

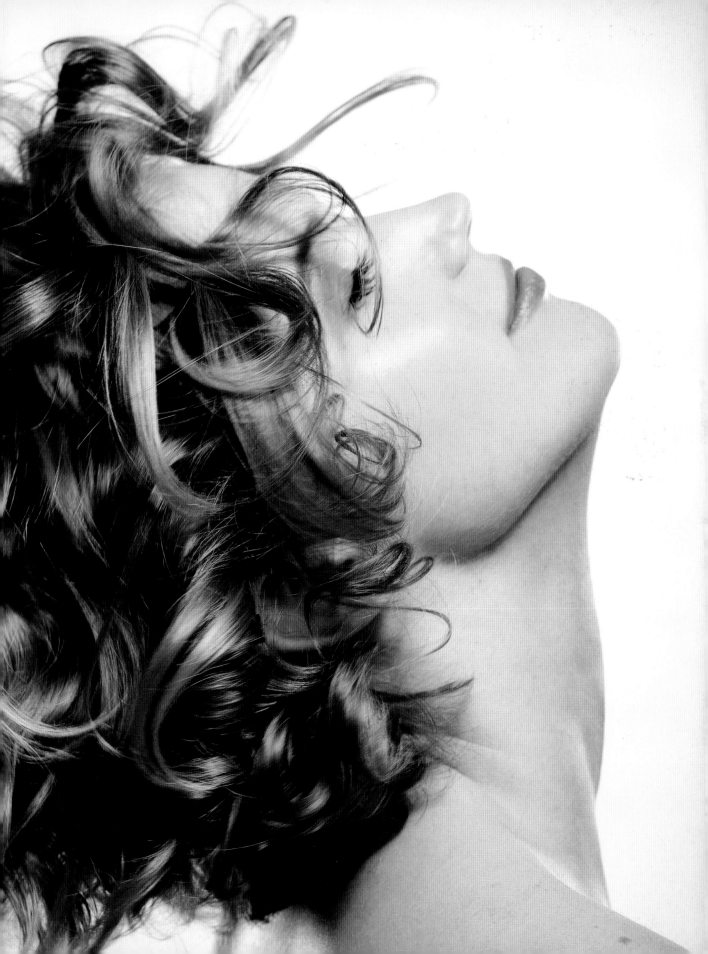

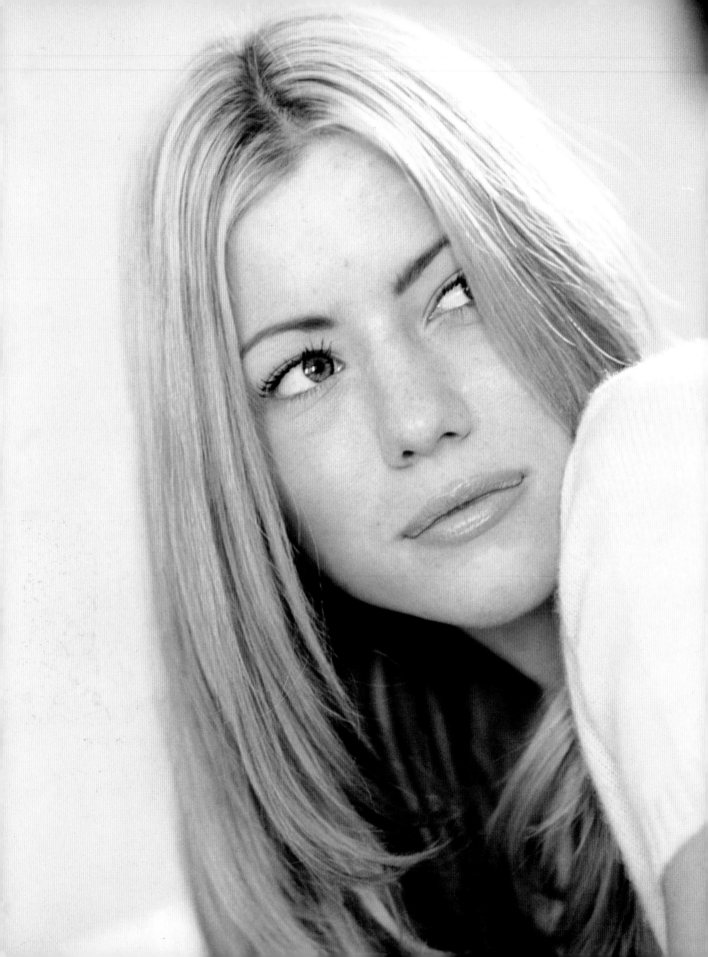

Your secret weapon: rollers

Good techniques and tools are critical for a problem we all face: how to get salon results at home.

A TRUE HASSLE It is not always obvious how to achieve the results of a successful salon blowout at home. The mirror gives you the image in reverse, and the round brush gets caught and refuses to go in the direction you want.

EXPRESS FORMAT The talented touch of a pro is difficult to imitate, but there is a trick that helps replicate the results: large Velcro rollers. This is the ideal rescue solution when you are styling hair at home before a party, for example.

Wrap your dry hair around the rollers, then spray lightly with hairspray and leave them in while you dress and do your makeup.

ADVICE FROM A STYLIST
Protective styling products, made to shield the cuticle from the heat of the blowdryer, must be used in the correct amounts. These products must also be distributed well and combed evenly through the hair.

Take the rollers out at the last minute, style your hair gently with your fingers, and smooth only the surface with a comb rather than a brush. Do not comb deep into the hair: If you do, you'll lose all the volume!

MIXED MEDIA (at right) Use rollers at the crown for maximum volume, then continue with a brush and blowdryer for the back and sides.

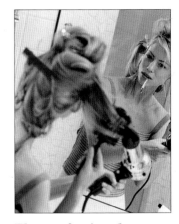

The professional method!
Work from roots to ends for perfect results.

The
reflective
effect,
the brazen
shine of hair
that's
totally
healthy

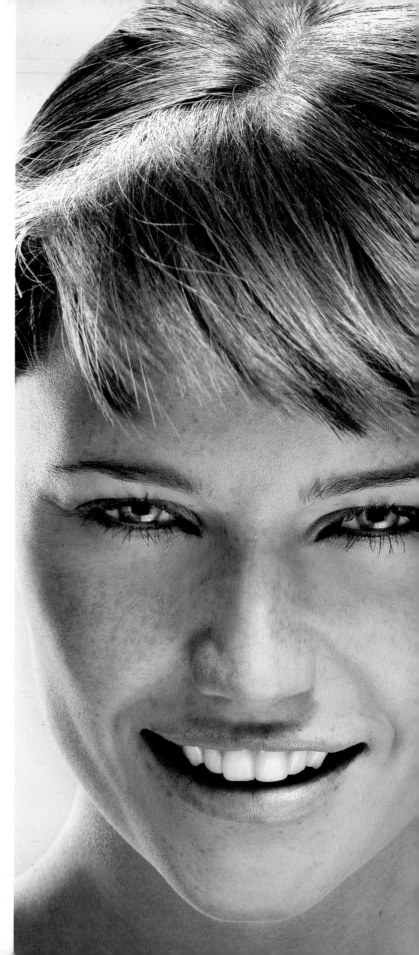

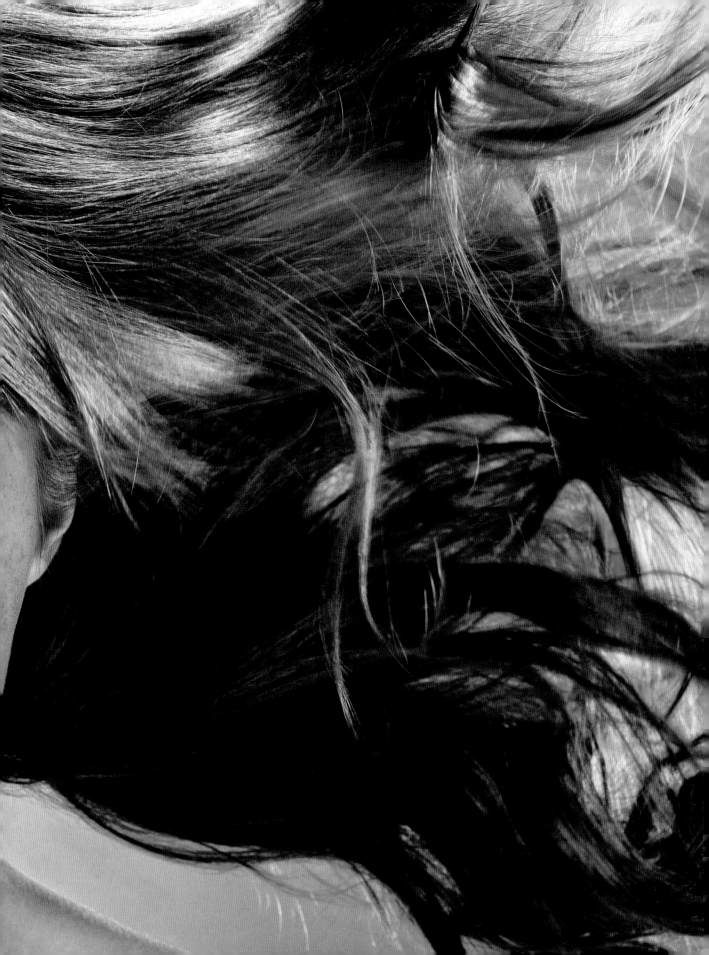

Check matte

Hair that shines all over is our number one demand—and rightly so! Silky luster is the most obvious sign of healthy hair.

ADVICE FROM A DERMATOLOGIST
Vitamins B5 and B8, sulfuric amino acids, essential fatty acids, extracts of vegetable oils: All provide a growth spurt for hair and nails!

Precious citrus:
Fruit acids ensure maximum shine: the reflective effect is the result of tightening the scales. They also have the benefit (similar to vinegar) of eliminating all traces of sediment deposited on hair by hard water, which dulls the fiber. These home remedies are very effective!

VOTE ANTI-DULL! Drab, matte hair is immediately perceived as unhealthy.

Shiny hair is the proof, not only that we pay attention to our appearance and that we take care of ourselves, but also that we have mastered the use of styling products (consider the difference between a synthetic "wet look" and soft, natural shine). Hair is like a tube, with more or less overlapping scales. The farther they are from the root, the more the scales lift and the less they shine. And these little surface imperfections are what prevent light from reflecting.

BEAUTY DIET Balanced nutrition (amino acids, essential fatty acids, vitamins, minerals, trace elements) is vital for the synthesis of keratin. Therefore, dieting often causes deficiencies in nutritional elements that are important for the beauty of hair, particularly essential fatty acids (present in vegetable oils), minerals, and oil-soluble vitamins. This explains why strict diets often cause hair to lose shine and become weak. On the other hand, excess fat in a diet can lead to an overproduction of sebum.

GLOSSY EFFECT You can also cheat and obtain the maximum effect in one step: a shine spray that coats the hair, creating the illusion of a halo of light.

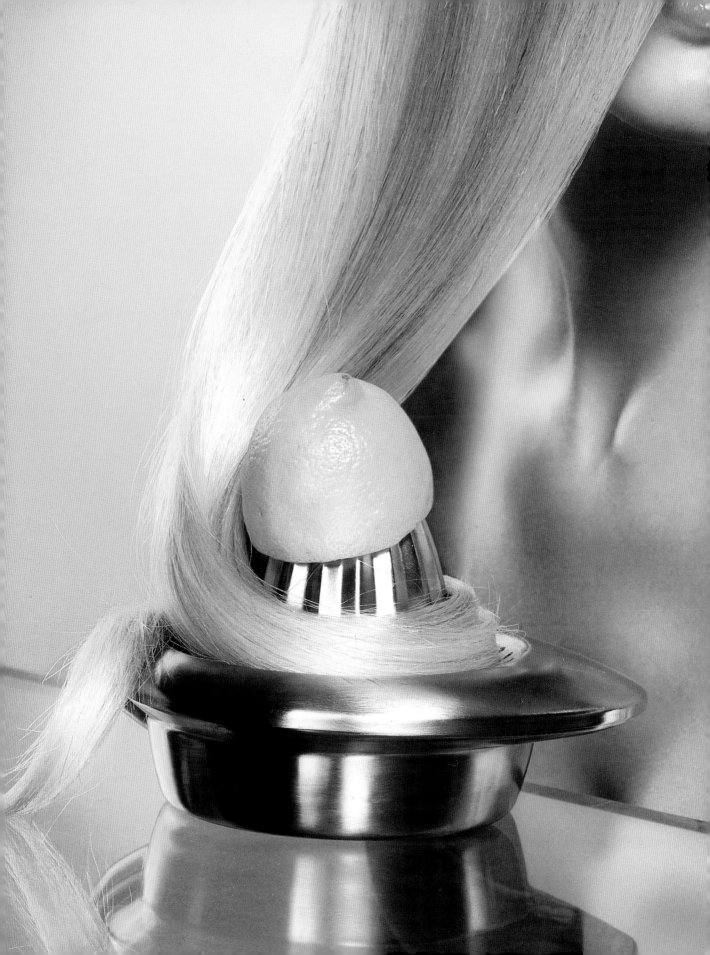

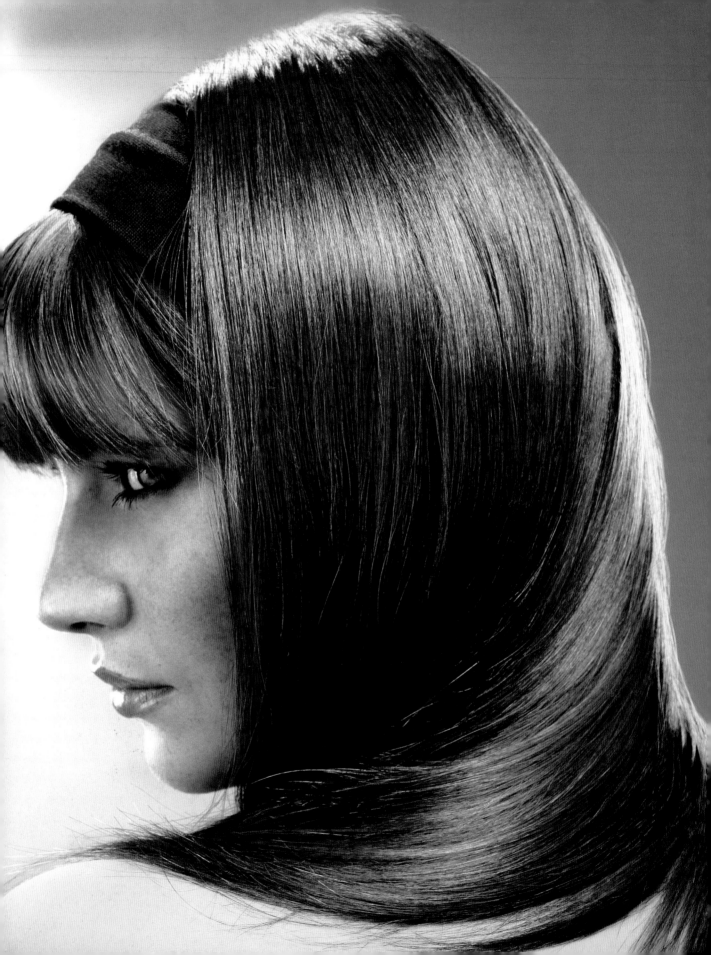

Sooo . . . sleek

Sleek hair is the most sought-after cosmetic result. The more we desire a natural look, the more we must use the advice of professional stylists and apply sophisticated products.

IMPECCABLY SLEEK SHINE happens in two steps: first, by "weighing down" hair to "deflate" it, and second, by nourishing it to **bring adhesion back to the scales** along the entire length of the strand. These steps ensure the most shine by bringing together both sleekness and perfect volume. This creates that sublime slow-motion fantasy where sleek, shiny hair slides and smoothly falls into place on either side of the face.

Here are some tricks to try:

AT HOME, use a softening shampoo, followed by a **hydrating mask** and shine solution. Blowdry your hair before straightening, according to your needs, with a flatiron (see side column) for shining results, but do not repeat this process too often if your hair is color-treated. And don't forget the heat-protective products!

AT THE SALON, smoothing treatments are incomparably effective, and you get a consultation as part of the deal!

ADVICE FROM A STYLIST
A ceramic flatiron is an essential ally to fans of impeccably sleek shine. Ceramic has the advantage of drying uniformly. You must remember, however, to allow it to cool completely before going over it again.

In-depth on volume

Fine hair has only one obsession: more volume! Here's what you need to make your dreams of fullness a reality.

To obtain the lift you covet, you need to start adding **body.** Beyond good nutrition, this involves bolstering your hair with leave-in conditioners, mousses, and styling products whose effects you will notice but whose presence you will not be able to see or feel. These types of products will give body back to even the flattest hair.

Volumizing gel: Apply to the roots of your hair and dry using a round brush.

Finishing spray: Spritz all over to put the final touches on your style.

THE WAVE OF ROLLERS: This is an ideal solution for those who are hopeless at blowdrying. Rollers today have nothing in common with the "sets" of the 1960s or your grandmother's curlers. Velcro rollers are the perfect way to finish doing your hair after you've used the appropriate styling products (spray or mousse), and then blowdry hair with your head flipped over (see page 43).

ADVICE FROM STYLIST BERNARD FRIBOULET
Four large rollers on top of the head is the professional stylist's trick for adding volume and avoiding the unsightly "hole" that divides the hair on the back of your head.

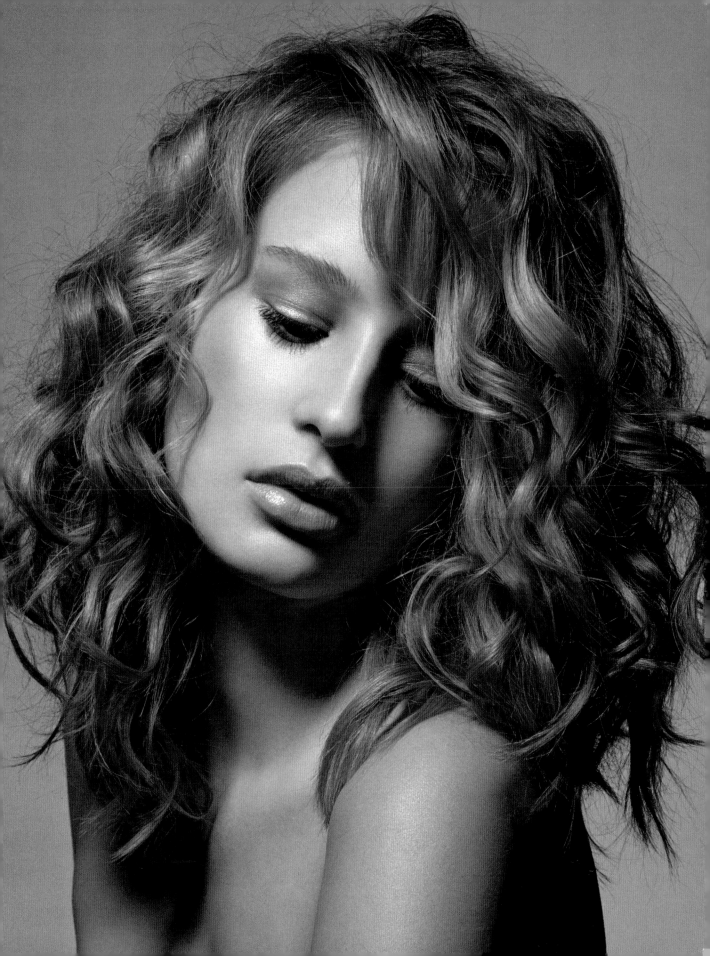

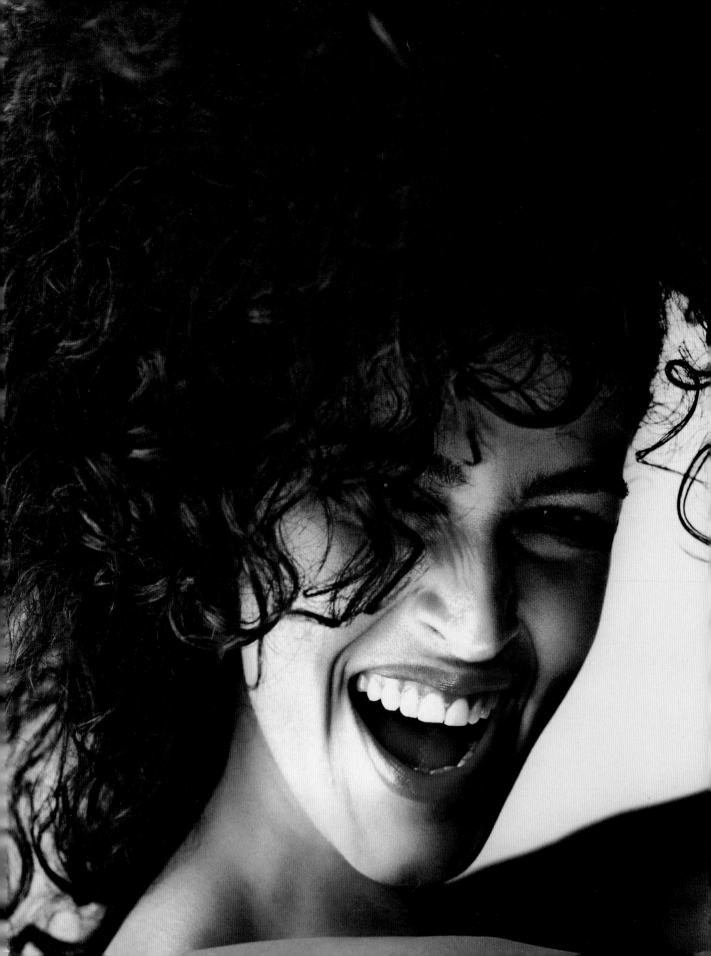

Curly perfection

Mastering unruly hair is the number one objective for those who are lucky enough to have natural curls but who spend their time (especially when it's humid outside) fighting frizz.

CONTROLLING CURLY HAIR Very curly hair has a dry texture because of its irregular surface—sebum distributes less evenly on curly hair than on straight. The insufficiently lubricated fiber has a tendency to be duller, and its lifted scales make it difficult to untangle. As a result, it shines less.

DO NOT GO SOFT The fuzzy, soft-focus effect is not flattering. You do not want to lose your ringlets, but rather define them and control the curl.

Undesirable frizz is very often located at the hairline and neck because the hair here is frequently finer, drier, and more exposed to bad weather, stress, strain, and pollution.

Anti-frizz and anti-humidity serums, invented to nourish curly hair without weighing it down, are perfect solutions.

ADVICE FROM A STYLIST
Why does humidity stimulate frizz? Hair is so thirsty that it absorbs the moisture in the air and, as a result, finds its natural shape. Even as you leave the salon after a blowout, your hair's true nature may take charge!

Sea, salt, and sun

The combination of UV rays, salt, and water creates a formidable cocktail. Here's how to avoid summer hair damage.

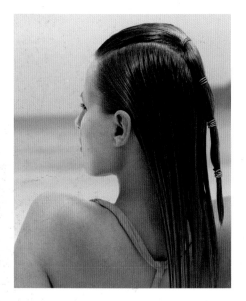

ADVICE FROM STYLIST BRUNO SILVANI

• Thoroughly coat hair with conditioners before swimming to protect it.

• In a pinch, if you have forgotten your special sun-protective product, do not hesitate to use a little bit of sunscreen on your hair!

THE EXPLOSIVE MIXTURE OF UV RAYS AND THE SUN is very harsh on hair. On the one hand, the resulting "summer blonde" can be gorgeous and can really complement slightly sunkissed skin, but on the other hand, it's a change from your natural color (and don't forget that certain delicate blondes can turn green thanks to chlorine).

Use preventive protection including specific oils, ultra-protective treatments, and nourishing shampoos, and be sure to give hair the extra attention it needs after exposure. All you have to do is touch your hair to realize that it needs a little finesse. In your hand, it will feel a bit more rough, almost thirsty.

APRÈS SUN, USE A "SHOCK" TREATMENT to repair it all! **Apply nutritive oil** a few hours before shampooing and leave hair wrapped in a towel. **Shampoo** your hair using a gentle formula and lukewarm water. **Apply a hair mask** over the entire length of the strand (starting about a half inch from the root) and allow it to sink in for about ten minutes. **Rinse thoroughly**, finishing with a splash of cool water to smooth out the scales on the shaft. To further protect hair, **allow it to air-dry** at least 50 percent before you use the dryer.

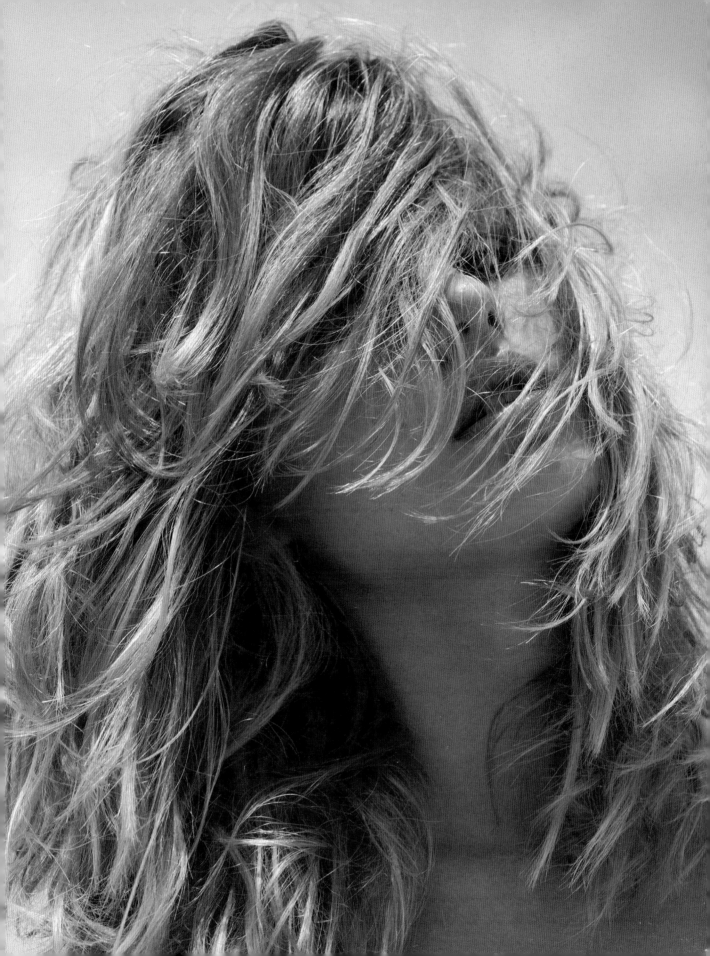

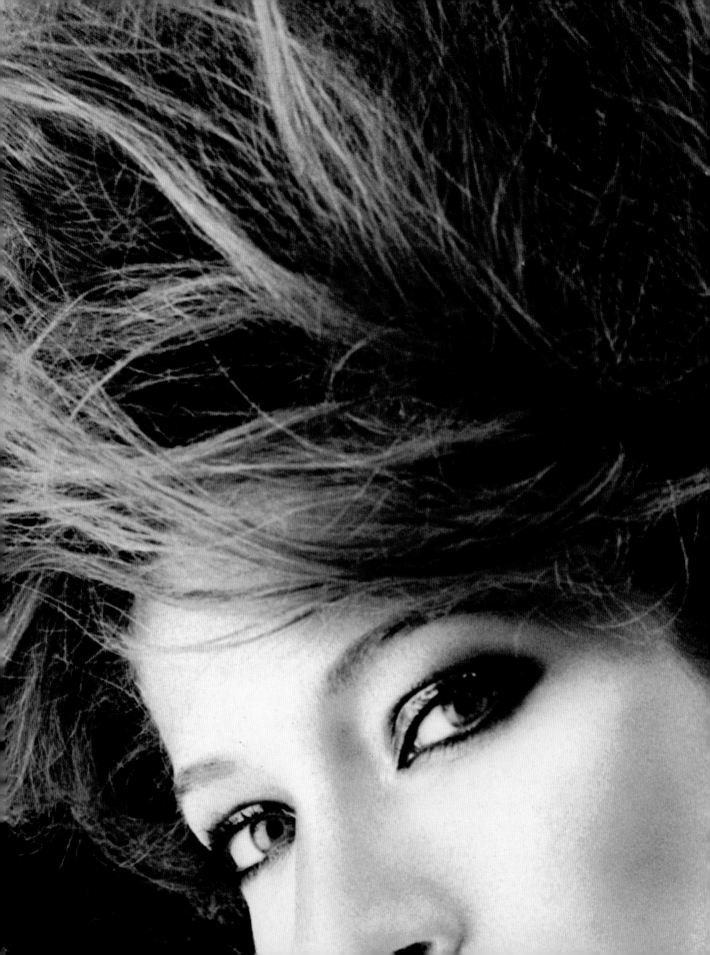

De-stress your tresses

Brittle, full of static, assaulted at every turn? Here's how to ease problems, detox your hair, and give damaged strands a few moments of peace.

STATIC Stop brushing, warm a bit of smoothing serum in your hands, and apply to hair. Static will no longer be a problem.

DAILY WASHING Use shampoo formulated for frequent use, and rinse in very warm water. This works much better than volumizing products.

CALM YOUR SCALP Your stylist has products and techniques for at-home hair masks that offer long-lasting shine.

DANDRUFF CONTROL We often forget that the scalp is part of the hair until we begin to experience discomfort and itching, the forerunners of dandruff. You must stop it in its tracks! Dandruff is caused by an **imbalance** in the natural microflora on the surface of the scalp. Dandruff (which is especially visible in long hair) is made up of cells on the scalp whose cycles have been disturbed—the part of the scalp that is of poor quality and is flaking off.

Although products have existed for a long time, today we are becoming much smarter about treating dandruff. No longer content to simultaneously ease the discomfort and erase the visible signs, we now seek to **re-establish the natural balance** of the scalp. Preventive logic leads to better results.

ADVICE FROM A RESEARCHER
Discomfort can also take the form of tightness, making you feel as though your scalp is a bit dry. Some shampoos have a hydrating element for the scalp, but can weigh down hair. Fortunately, all shampoos today respect the scalp, and we no longer have the harsh detergents that can cause irritation.

Counteracting hair loss and signs of age

We all want eternally young hair, but it cannot last forever. There are many reasons for hair loss, but thankfully, there are solutions.

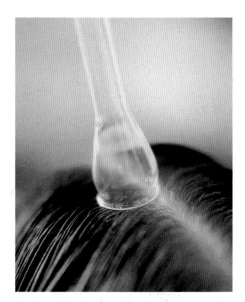

ADVICE FROM A PSYCHOLOGIST

From disappointment in love to powerful emotions, all types of temporary crises can take their toll on hair and cause it to fall out. It is difficult to make a direct association, however, since three months or so usually elapse between the stressful event and the resulting hair loss. Nonetheless, the relationship is undeniable. (Source: *Les Cheveux et la Vie,* Dr. Danièle Pomey-Rey)

EACH HAIR FOLLICLE LIVES FOR TWENTY-FIVE SUCCESSIVE GENERATIONS thanks to a generous dose of estrogen, helping to protect women from baldness. Men, on the other hand, are the first to lose their hair because of high levels of testosterone. Nonetheless, there's no denying that hair loss also happens to women. The first sign is if you begin to notice loose hairs, rather than clumps (no need to panic—significant losses are actually less serious). There are many causes, from lack of iron and amino acids to the stresses of styling. Talk to your doctor or stylist about what action to take.

A BIT OF HELP Anti-hair-loss cures treat the symptoms very effectively while improving hair quality. From daily shampooing, which lifts your spirits at the same time, to coloring your hair (which causes no harm), to specialized massages for a poorly irrigated scalp, there are ways to get things back on course.

WITH AGE, hair becomes more and more strained, starts to thin out, is harder to style, and is drier to the touch. If hair loss is present, an imperfect covering of the scalp causes aesthetic problems. New lines of products and nutritional supplements can help stimulate the hair and give it body.

HAIR EXTENSIONS can also fill in the gap while you are waiting for your own hair to grow in again.

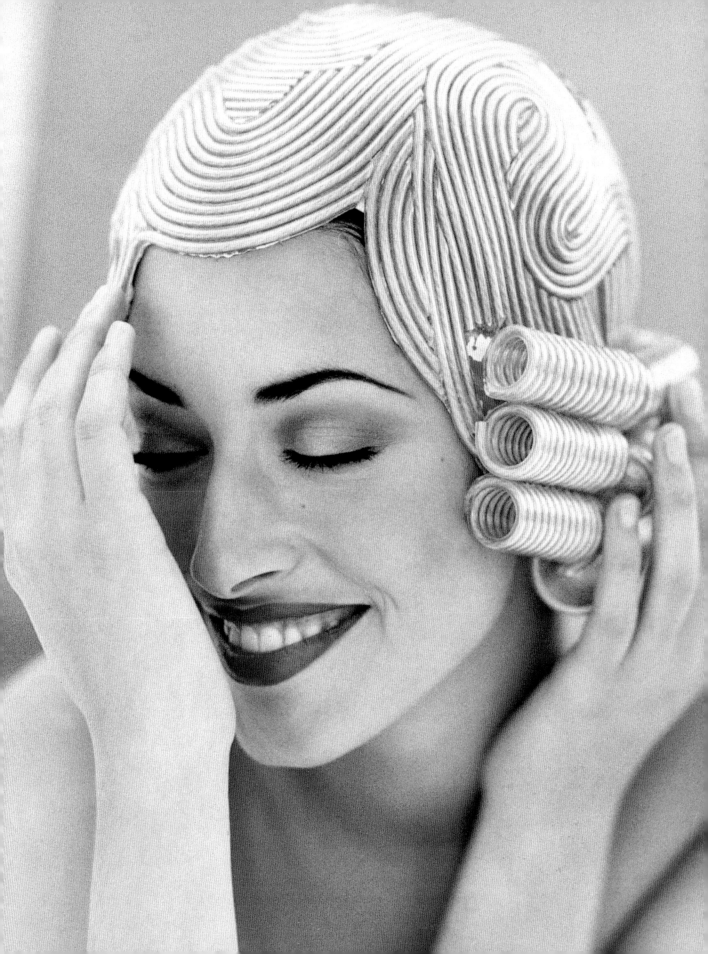

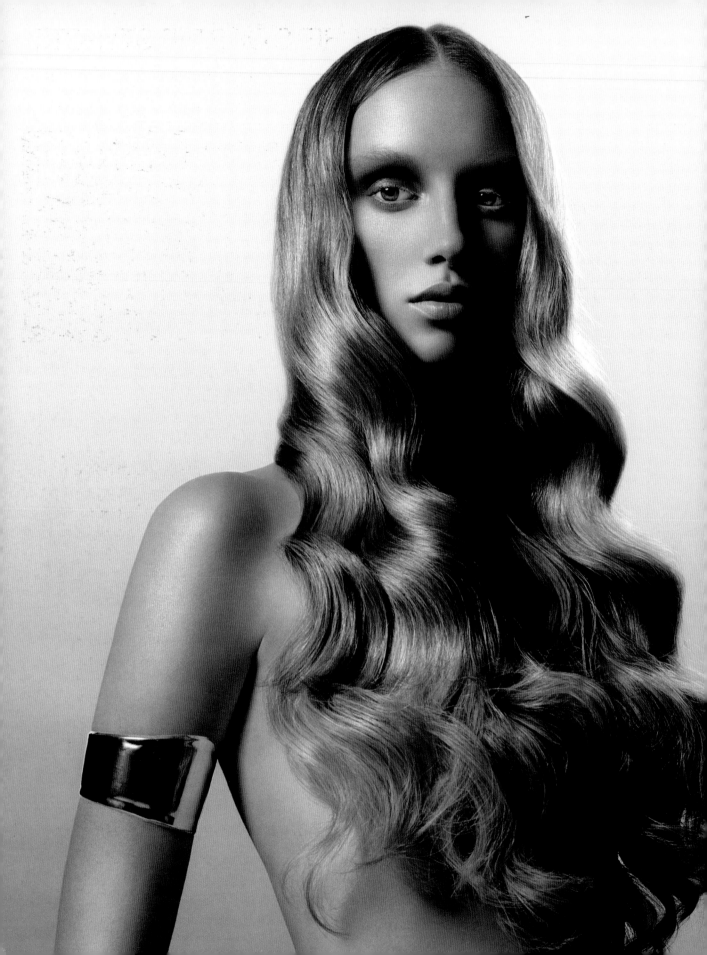

Grégory Kaoua

Artistic Director
L'Oréal Professionnel

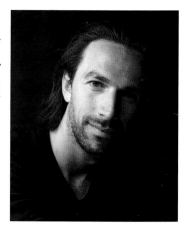

This young master—now a favorite of beauty companies and great photographers—discovered his love of beautiful things early, which helped set the course for his career. He has completely refined the world of hair photography by creating luxurious images that transform hair and give it a never-before-seen luster. For Kaoua, it's all about being in the moment.

"Today it is no longer about 'doing your hair,' no longer a matter of imposing a style. There is only one trend— what you desire!"

I have wanted this career since I was five. As early as third grade, I wanted to begin training in hair-dressing. Early on, though, I was disappointed because it was not the artistic world I'd expected. But, this is no longer the case today: In the past five or six years, salons have taken a turn. The artistic level is higher, and there is a clear connection to fashion and creativity—with the places that tell a story.

WE NO LONGER GO TO THE SALON JUST TO GET A TRIM!

I looked up French styling legend Odile Gilbert and went to see her at her studio. Her agent called me for my first fashion show with Chanel, which was a tremendous shock! Then one encounter changed my life: I met Clovis, a hair stylist with a true vision. He taught me to distort classical foundations, make them my own, modernize them. He helped me develop a certain look. I left everything behind to start over and become his assistant. My wife was extremely supportive and accepted that I was living my passion. I spent day in and day out with the master, carrying his equipment—two years of intense work.

▶

An incredible cascade of waves gives a Hollywood look that's updated and modern. They are slightly offbeat and original: instead of beginning at the shoulder, they start higher up.

"I love the double take: when you don't immediately notice that a woman has electric blue hair!"

It's all about feeling. You are not shown, like in cooking, how to prepare a sauce. No, you must love hair and what it does, watch how to manipulate it, and learn how to construct an image. A tiny subtlety, a slight movement, something ephemeral, a particular angle, can translate into a unique moment.

I've done unbelievable sessions for the most famous magazines. As a result of working with the most beautiful women in the world—Helmut Newton models, for example—your eye sharpens. When Clovis helped me understand there was nothing more for him to teach me, his agent Aurélien took me on as a solo stylist.

I TRULY LOVE BEAUTY—WITH STRIKING, DISTINCTIVE HAIR

I cut the proverbial cord and began my career with L'Oréal, working on my own hair research, and selling the product line. Thanks to my hard work, the company put its trust and confidence in me.

Kérastase was my first line of styling products. I was their adviser, testing products in the salon and helping to refine them. I worked on the designs, the models. I had the opportunity to be in artistic fusion with the artistic director.

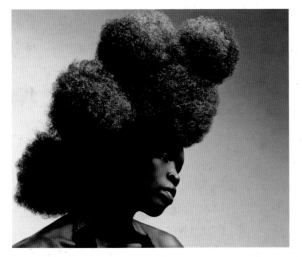

THE VERY FIRST KÉRASTASE IMAGE launched a new vision. It was a girl with tangled up hair, extreme volume, all while being incredibly beautiful. This was truly my talent, and I designed it and created it. This image marked a true shift, including in the United States, combining a very luxurious image with an international, elite, spa type of feel.

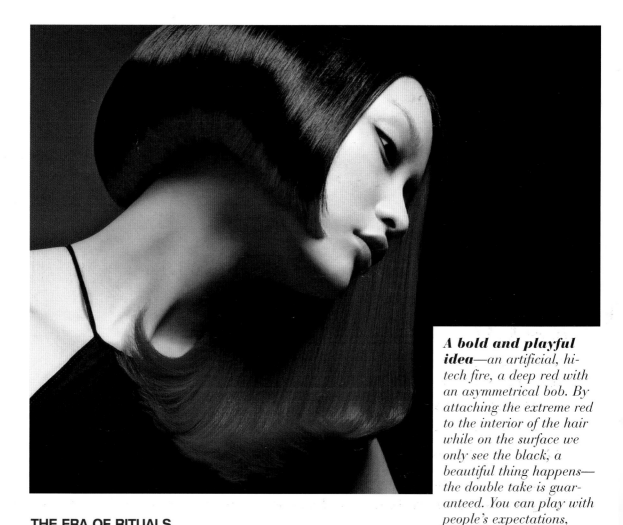

A bold and playful idea—*an artificial, hitech fire, a deep red with an asymmetrical bob. By attaching the extreme red to the interior of the hair while on the surface we only see the black, a beautiful thing happens— the double take is guaranteed. You can play with people's expectations, even at 50, by replacing the red with honey blonde, for example.*

THE ERA OF RITUALS

TODAY 70 PERCENT OF WOMEN HAVE COLORED OR HIGHLIGHTED HAIR. We are no longer in the era of the cut, but that of cared-for, healthy hair, luxurious in the Hermès sense, not ostentatious but refined. You can have any cut or style, so long as it is beautiful and voluminous. There are products that work well for all hair types, but there are also products that are adapted for fine hair. We're moving almost toward nanotechnology and becoming very specialized. It's not about marketing, it's about what is pleasing; you tell a beautiful story, make a beautiful image—and most importantly, the product works.

WHAT ARE THE MOST IMPORTANT TIPS? With this range, the products are powerful and ultra-nourishing—you don't simply wash your hair, you use shampoo as a cure. Taking vitamins for a month is the same as using our shampoo and after-shampoo treatments. If you find that your hair is soft, for example, you must not exceed the treatment time or your hair will become tired, lifeless, oversaturated. You should switch back and forth between two or three shampoos and conditioners throughout the year. It is very important to choose your ▶

"This is haute couture for the hair: if you own a Dior dress, you don't throw it in the washing machine!"

products based on the nature of your hair, your way of life, and the environment—if you live in Paris, your hair will become oily more quickly than if you live on the Côte d'Azur.

Also important: Before and after coloring your hair, do not forget to nourish it. Taking the extra step changes everything. The color will last longer, and hair will be healthier and better able to absorb the color. (Similarly, overly damaged hair will not take color evenly from roots to ends.) If you nourish it, your color won't become dull after two weeks, and it will stay shiny. If a woman wants truly beautiful color, she must take steps to care for it. Colored hair requires a bit of extra effort. If you own a beautiful Dior dress, you don't throw it in the washing machine!

I ADORE COLOR! Rosselli of L'Oréal Professionnel asked me to work on Matrix, Majirel, Luo. I love results that make people do a double take more than anything. I don't like anything showy, an assault of extreme colors. A red-blue-green look serves only to shock. It's much more playful and fun if you notice after five minutes that you are speaking with a woman who has a hint of electric blue in her hair—that is pure sophistication.

HAIR EXTENSIONS—A TRUE REVOLUTION! It's so amazing to have beautiful, thick hair immediately, to be able to play with length. At a stylist show, I had a simple lock of extensions, and I ended with incredible volume. You can do anything with them!

You can keep hair extensions in for two or three months, and because the keratin combinations are much finer, you can barely detect them. And you can wash your hair without a problem. The only drawback: they're still very expensive.

WHAT IS CUTTING EDGE is determined by certain fashion stylists! But I believe there is only one trend—your desire! It's great to be in style, but don't impose a hairstyle that is not your own. You'll be in fashion for ten days and be completely depressed afterwards. For example, "the bowl cut" or "all fringed" or, having gotten a ratty haircut, saying "the stylist does what he wants, he's such an artist!".

No, I am against that notion; we are not artists, but artisans, and I say that loud and clear. You must have **a true dialogue with your stylist.** This is becoming more and more acceptable and common practice, thankfully. With magazines, fashion shows that are accessible to everyone, the Internet, women genuinely have a ton of information: you know what you want.

▶

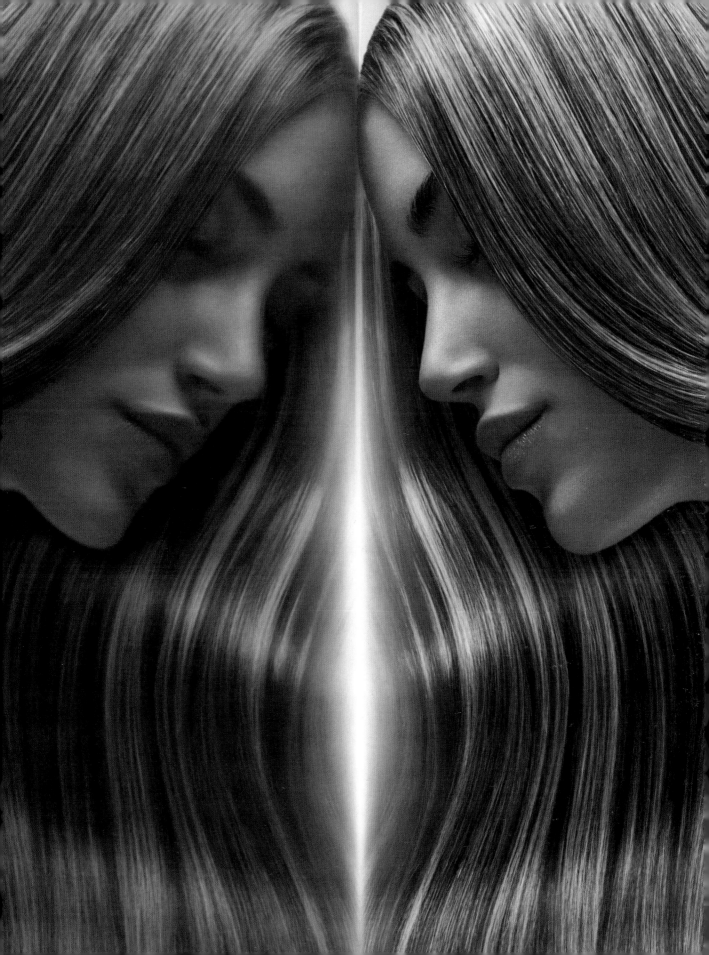

"Extreme heights: the work of an artisan from sketch to image, in artistic fusion!"

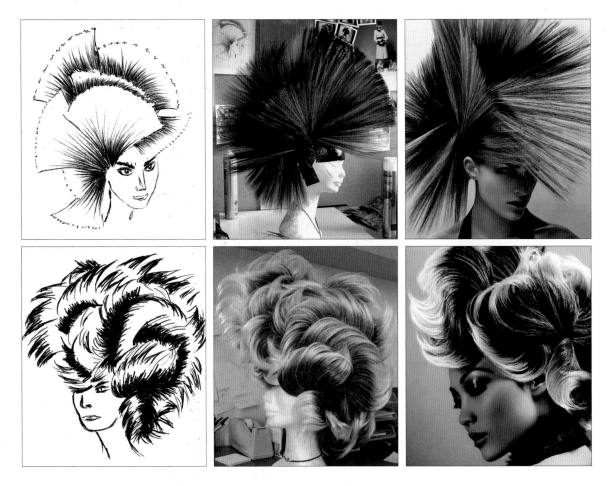

THE WORK OF AN ARTISAN, for the L'Oréal Professionel campaign (above). I was responsible for everything from the sketches to the final advertising image. This was not a montage: It was done in a studio and required the creation of 200 locks. It was a true puzzle, built piece by piece and representing several days of work. I love unexpected changes in plans—what you thought you would use as bangs can be used at the nape!

NUDE COLORS (at right) A subtle shading and blending of colors into one another, from chocolate brown to dark red. The colors designed the style, allowing the most extreme play on tones.

I do not like uniform colors, I love to play with reflections and materials—highlights, subtle shading from roots to tips, from golden blonde to ash blonde.

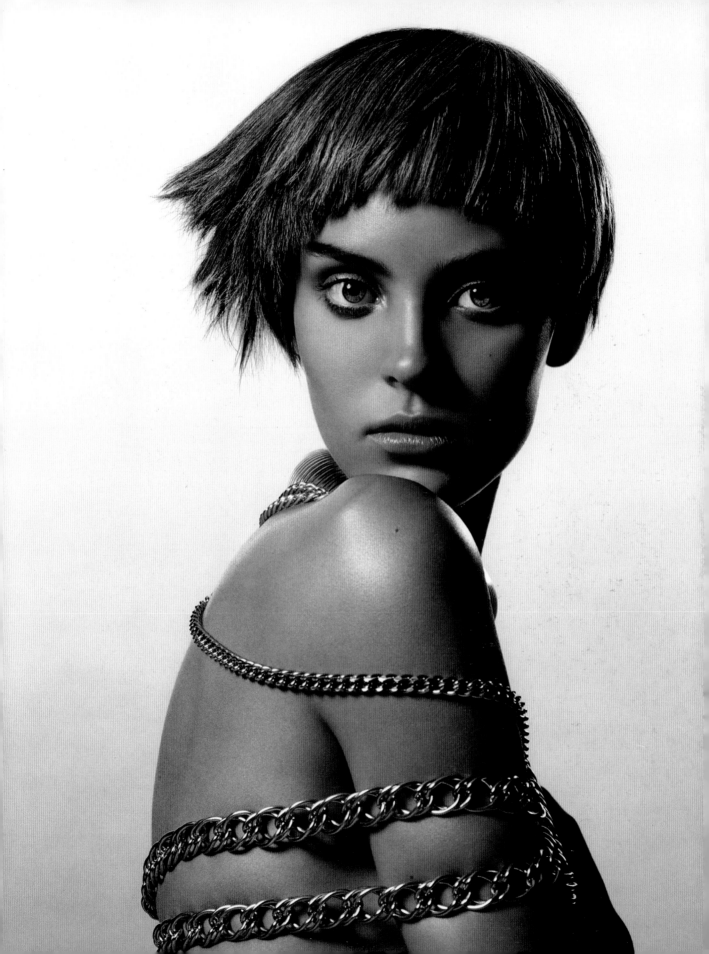

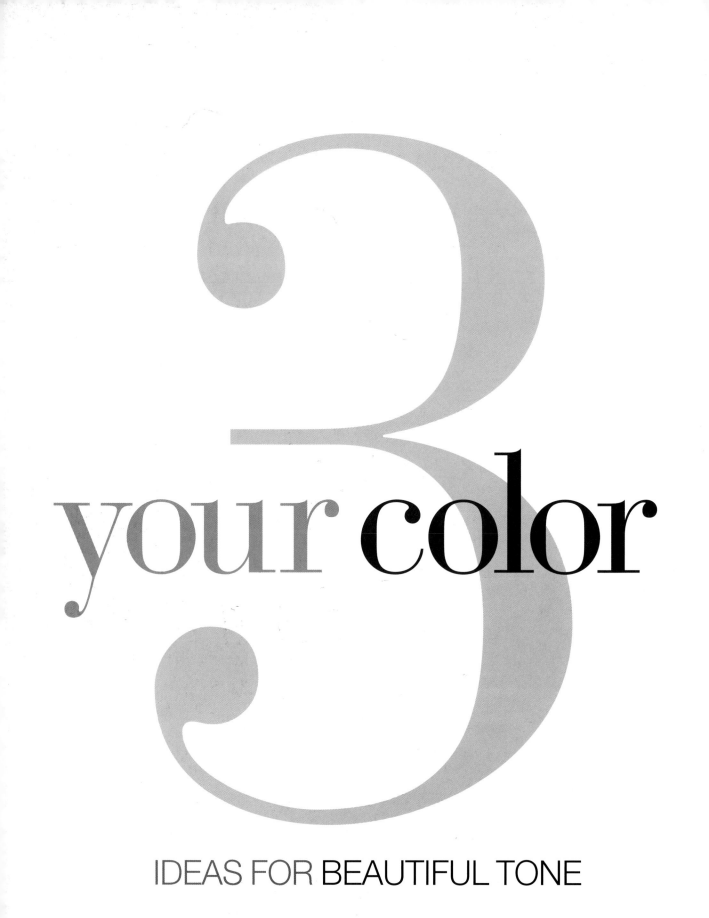

3 your color

IDEAS FOR BEAUTIFUL TONE

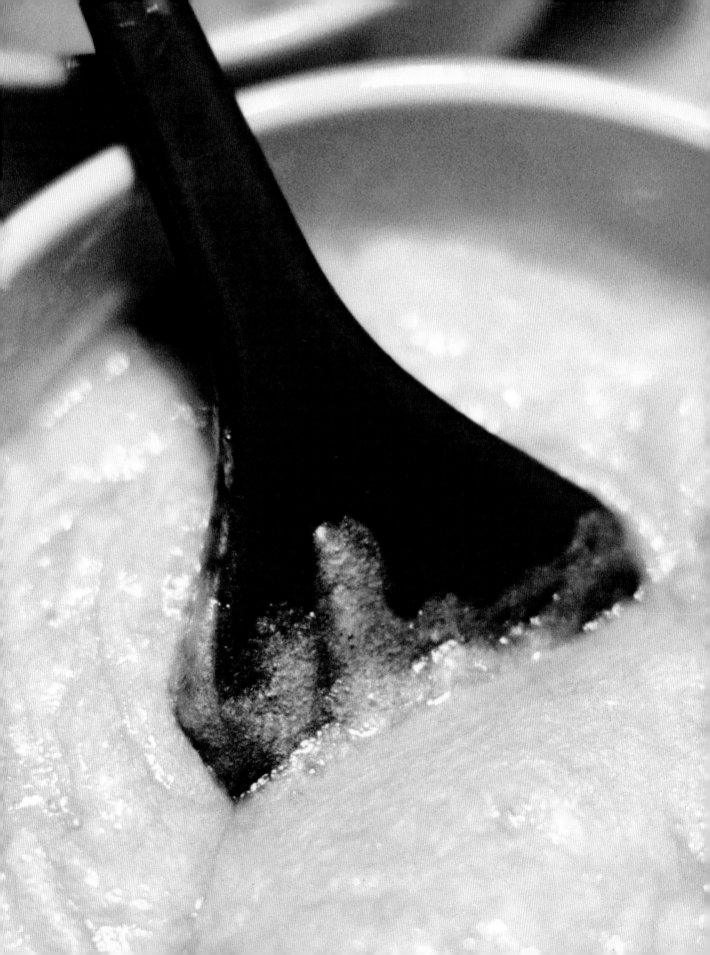

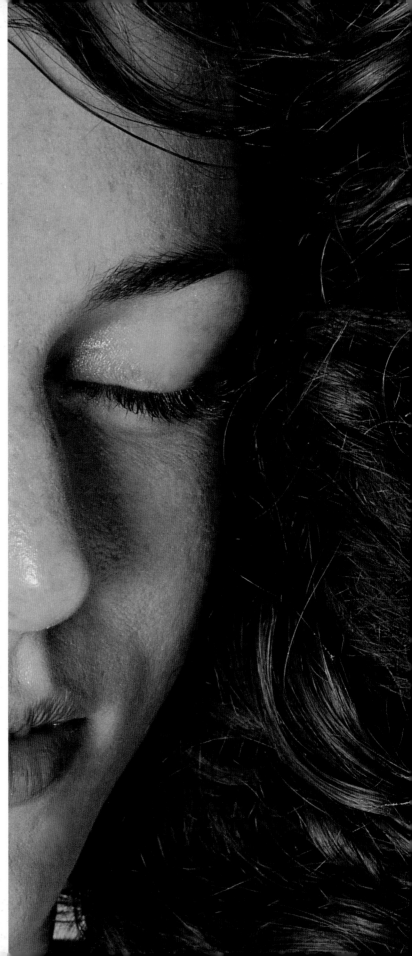

Find
your mode of
expression
to bring out
your personality

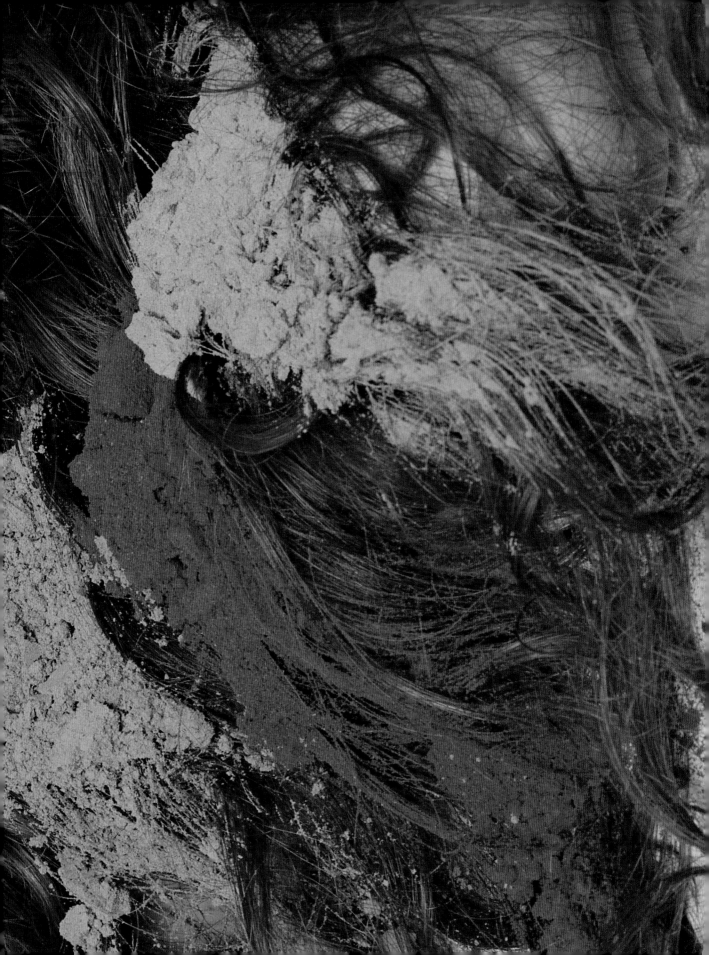

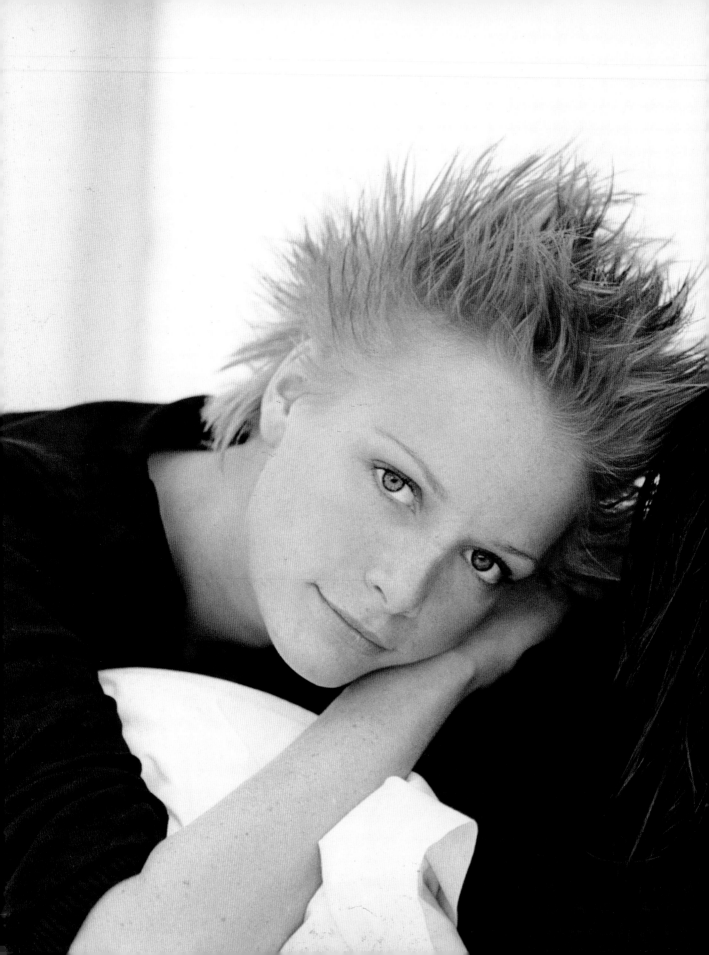

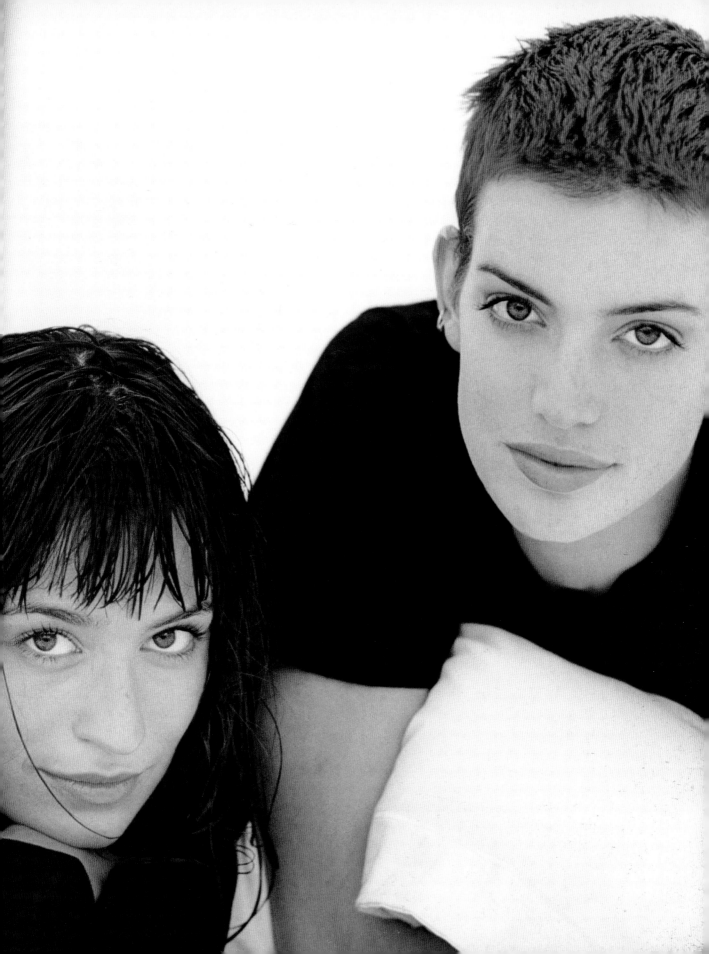

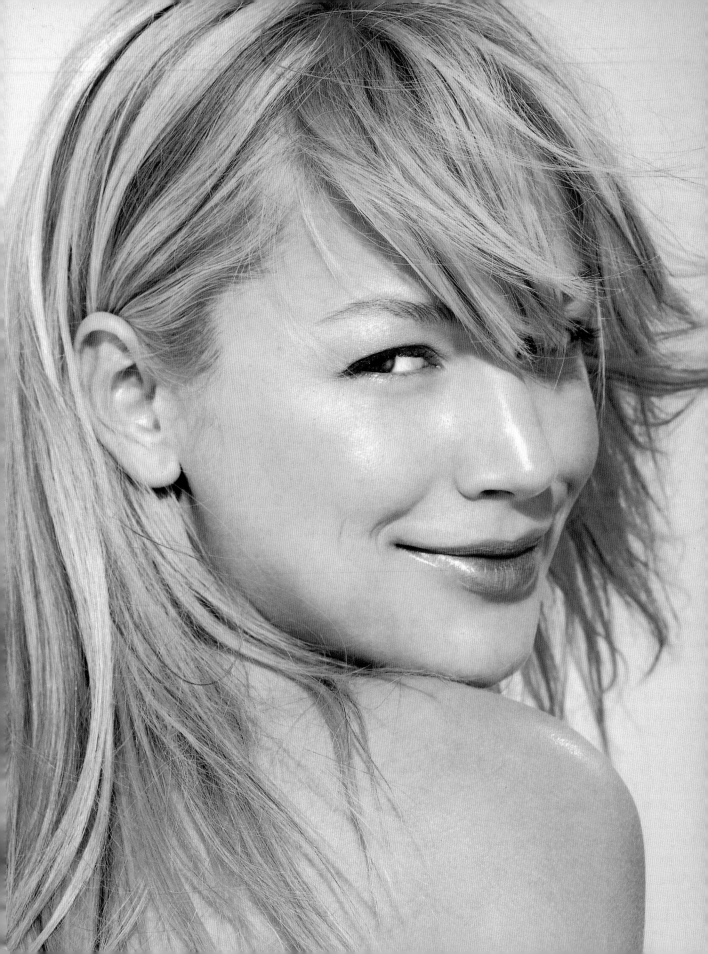

Blonde: the secret weapon of seduction

Blonde has always been the golden yardstick for classical beauty. But it has also seen a revolution in all its shades.

ALWAYS MYTHICAL, blonde casts you in full light, although paradoxically it will never be as shiny as darker hair. From angelic lightness to *femme fatale,* from Marilyn Monroe and Brigitte Bardot to Sharon Stone, Catherine Deneuve to Madonna, blonde hair has always symbolized a certain image of femininity, one that is sometimes also criticized. Today this color is available in a range of subtle shades.

Baby blonde is reserved for people with delicate complexions and light skin. It lends a childhood innocence to the face, evoking the beach and the sun.

Avoid going too light, or you will wash out your complexion and your face.

Wheat blonde begins with light undertones and blends in darker shades with personalized highlights.

Then there are **warmer shades,** such as dark golden blonde, caramel, hazelnut, honey, and more contrasting tones. With these, always stay one or two shades lighter or darker than the base.

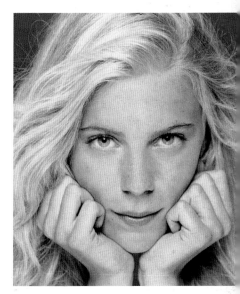

ADVICE FROM STYLIST BERNARD FRIBOULET
Women today refuse strict rules and do not want to be slaves to frequent salon visits because of obvious roots. The solution? Switch to honey or Venetian blonde, which gives it a youthful glow and requires less maintenance.

Red: the secret weapon of seduction

Red hair is finally now recognized for its true value.

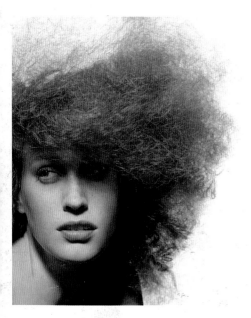

A FLAMBOYANCE THAT HAS COME DOWN THROUGH THE AGES, red hair is associated with romanticism and a fiery temper. In reality, whether you are born with red hair or you dye your hair red, there is no more striking combination for people who have fair skin.

Unlike other shades, red frequently requires a uniform coloring (but this is not an absolute rule). Above all, though, red hair needs shine and depth.

Artificial red is very susceptible to everyday stresses: Color-care shampoo and styling products used together are the only way to preserve its fire.

Red is in! Red, the archetypal bold color, has made a tremendous breakthrough. What's next?

Colorists can dare to do anything, including undertones of green, copper, and brown. But they are also experimenting with plum and antique rose.

ADVICE FROM COLORIST RODOLPHE

I am against uniform color, even for redheads. A few sections of dark chocolate in a shocking red will help it stand out even more. You must create volume, shape, and contrast.

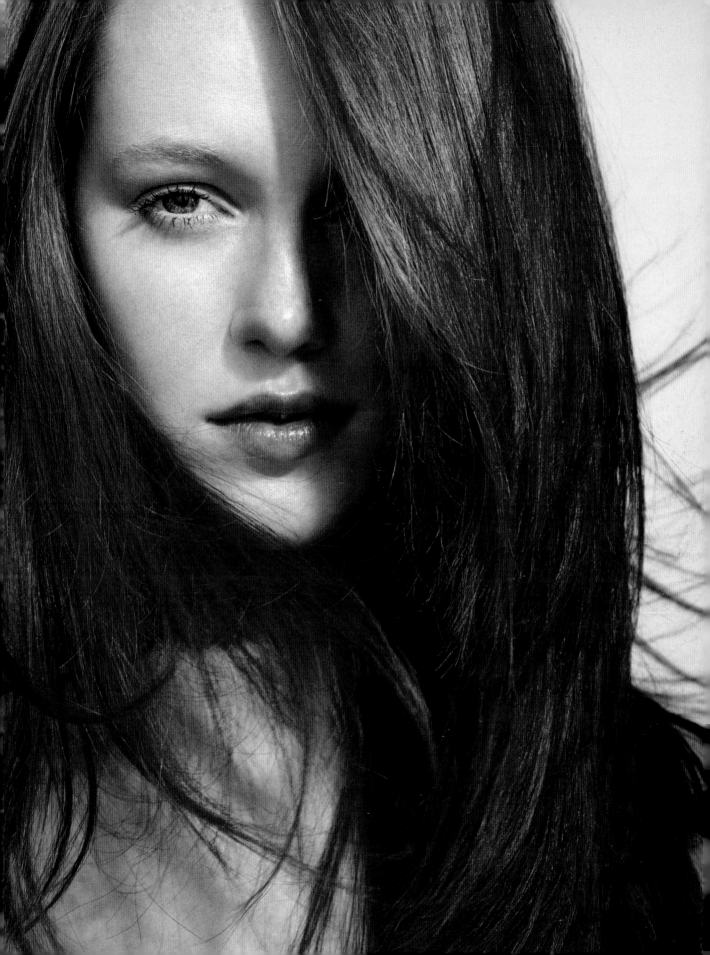

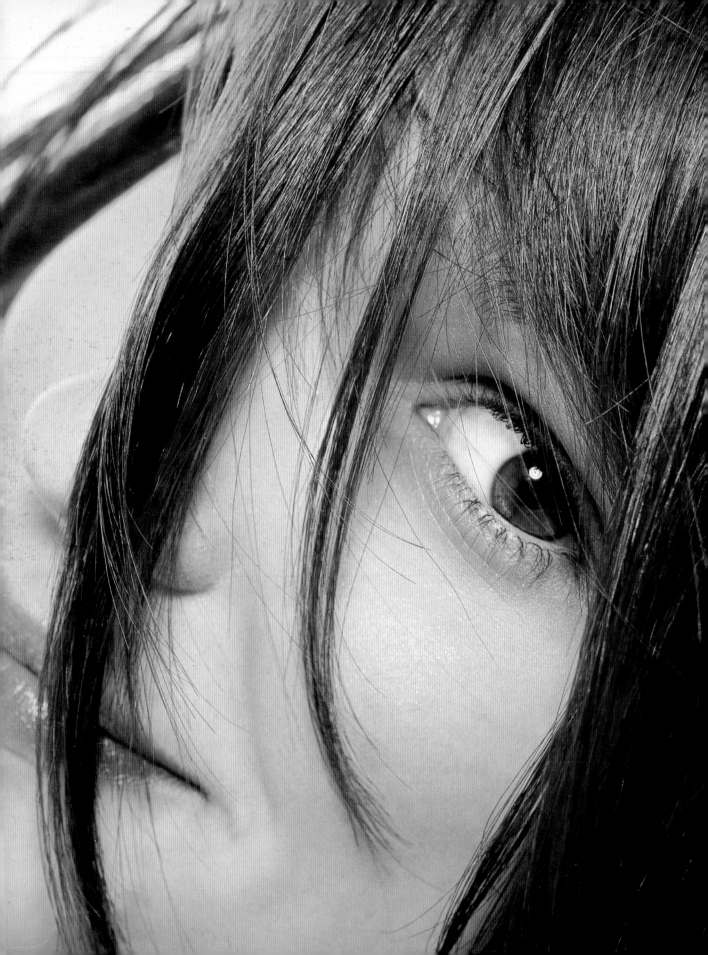

Chestnut: the secret weapon of seduction

We have yet to see all the surprises this color has in store. Chestnut celebrates its great return with quiet sophistication—personality required.

CHESTNUT WITHOUT DISAPPOINTMENT Hazelnut, frosted brown, chocolate, shortbread cookie—this is a gourmet vocabulary to rekindle our love of the most widespread, but also the most misunderstood, hair color.

Deep and luminous, chestnut also blossoms into shades of copper and mahogany. It has one absolute priority: to emerge from the shadows. To play up chestnut, add highlights to create a sunkissed look, which is not, contrary to popular belief, reserved for blondes.

Bring out the best by playing with the spectrum of colors: from basic chestnut, you can lighten a few sections or introduce darker tones at your whim, taking into account your complexion and eye color.

Be aware that straight and curly, long and short hair do not absorb color in the same way, and only a colorist can decide what works best for yours.

These shades look great on everyone:
• Coppers
• Dark browns

These shades are best for fair skin and light eyes:
• Ash browns
• Classic browns

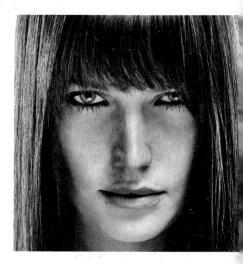

ADVICE FROM STYLIST JOHN NOLLET
So long as it shimmers with multiple and varied reflections, all while remaining within the same tonality, chestnut hair will flatter your complexion. This color is superb for medium-length hair or long hair that is layered, as it takes on all its depth.

Brunette: the secret weapon of seduction

More than ever before, brunettes are standing out. From medium shades to the darkest black, anything goes and beauty is guaranteed.

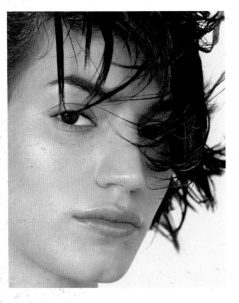

RAVEN BLACK WITH REFLECTIONS OF MIDNIGHT BLUE is recommended if you already have a darker complexion. It illuminates lighter eyes.

What personality! Dark colors go well with all hairstyles but work especially well with stylized, extremely precise cuts. All types of bobs look particularly great.

Embellishing brown hair: Brown and dark chocolate warm pale complexions.

Ash brown and copper help to tone down ruddy complexions.

Natural chestnuts will turn into pretty browns, but if you have light hair, it will be difficult to get good results with the darkest shades in this spectrum.

Adding highlights to lighter shades will offer the look of texture.

Beware: Hair gradually gets lighter from roots to ends.

To help maintain good tone between colorings, there is an entire category of shampoos that deposit color and help give hair back its vigor and depth.

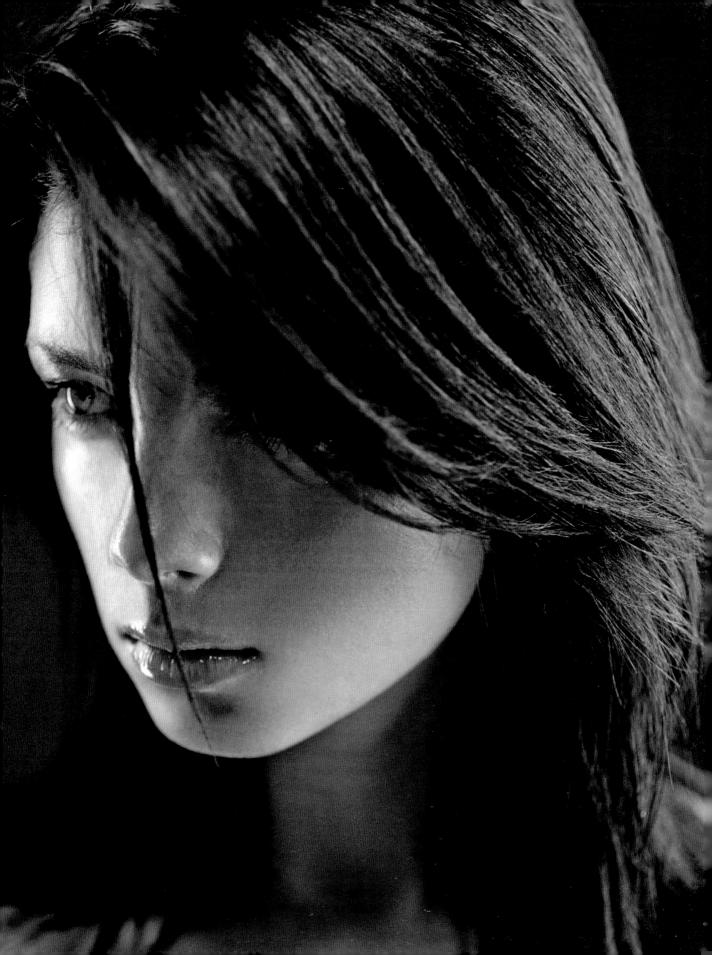

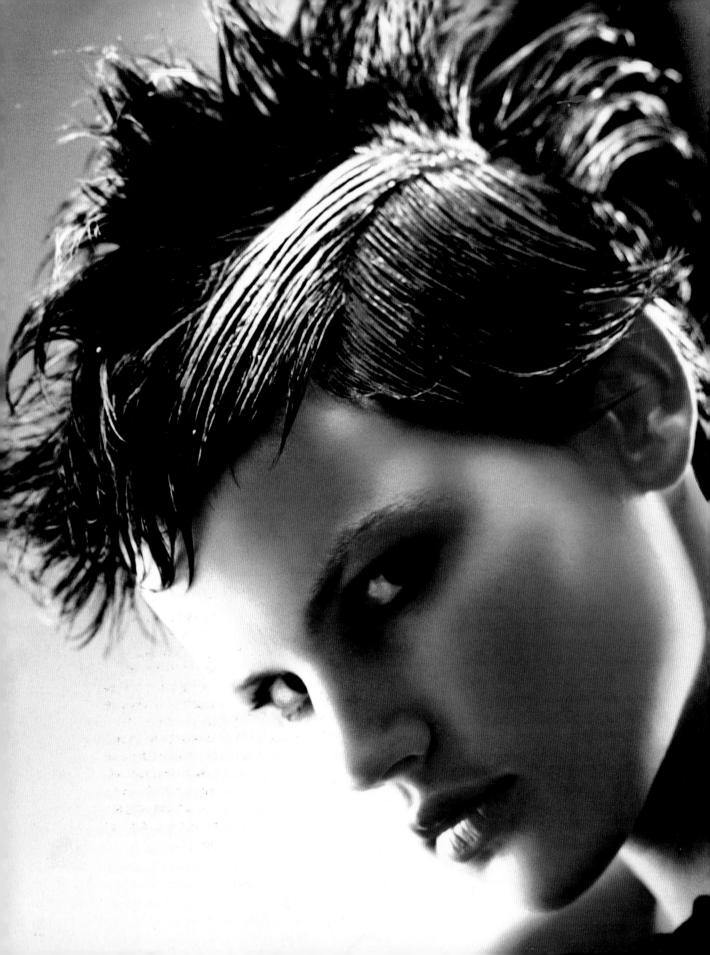

Color to fit your mood

Today, nothing is more natural than coloring your hair. The proof? Over 70 percent of women have done it. A new generation of products is helping to ease any lingering fears of coloring, systematically integrating the notion of healthy hair into their formulation.

DOWN WITH UNIFORMITY! We want color, now more than ever! But we want hair coloring that blends harmoniously into a natural tonality, not something uniform. We want to do away with the helmet effect and monochromatic highlights: we want contrasts to better capture light, play with reflections and create the illusion of volume. Not only do we now have incredibly rich palettes, but stylists are happy to develop combinations that result in original colors, re-creating a perfect natural look.

This is an extremely technical approach, which explains why coloring remains the quintessential professional technique. And while half of all coloring is done at home, a stylist always has the magic touch for the best possible results.

AN UNEXPECTED LEVEL OF CARE Today the act of coloring is an act of hair care. More than simply covering grays or getting the color you want, it also requires improving hair health. Coloring products are becoming much milder, with gentler formulas that smell good and make your hair healthier. Surprisingly, many women find that their hair has exceptional texture and shine after coloring!

ADVICE FROM COLORIST RODOLPHE
As unique as a fingerprint, hair color is made up of thousands of shades. How do you choose, when hundreds of possibilities exist in each color palette? Here is the absolute test: A successful color must be beautiful not only in flattering light, but also first thing in the morning when you wake up!

Coloring:
How it works

Thanks to new technology, products are becoming more and more gentle and easier to use, but coloring your hair is never entirely harmless.

ADVICE FROM COLORIST RODOLPHE

You should space colorings so they are enjoyable and do not feel like a chore. While you cannot prevent your hair from growing, you can make the regrowth appear less linear, less visible.

To avoid mild discomfort, try applying permanent coloring on unwashed hair. (The natural oils in your scalp will provide a protective barrier.) With oily hair, permanent coloring will be beneficial because it temporarily reduces sebaceous secretions.

TWO FAMILIES OF COLORING

1 Temporary coloring: This type coats the hair with colored substances and will fade after several shampoos. It does not change the **natural melanin,** because it stays on the outside of the cortex without going to the heart of the hair shaft. Temporary coloring is the perfect solution for those first grays.

2 Permanent coloring or oxidation coloring: Developed to cover a larger quantity of gray hair, permanent coloring contains substances that bring about a chemical reaction, allowing dyes to penetrate to the heart of the hair fiber and change the color of hair.

Classic oxidation coloring: With this type of permanent coloring, a blend of coloring products and oxidants penetrate the hair to strip it of color (eliminating part or all of the natural melanin) before coloring it again in the chosen shade.

Tone-on-tone oxidation coloring: This type of permanent hair coloring penetrates the hair fiber and deposits around the cortex. The coloring does not lighten the fiber. Instead of modifying the natural color, it superimposes itself transparently. It enhances your original shade, so hair remains in the same tonal family, but just a bit darker.

HOW LONG WILL IT LAST? Over time, and as a result of repeated washings, highlights will fade and the color will lose its brilliance. Our number one wish? To preserve the intensity of hair's color between colorings!

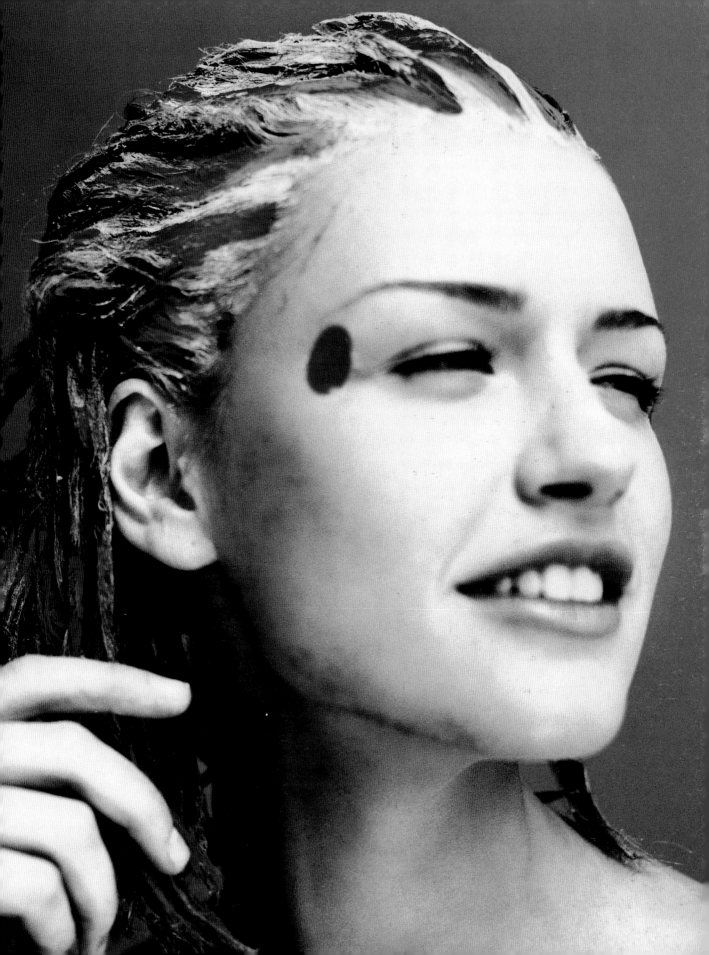

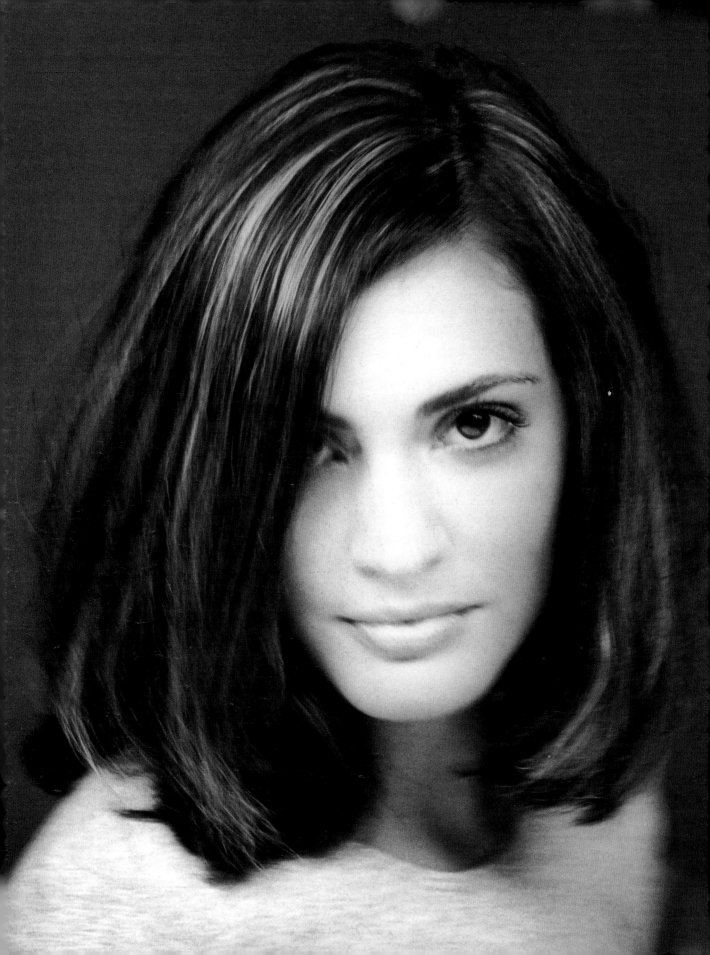

Gray hair: the game of hide and seek

Accept it or conceal it? The loss of pigmentation in hair, which usually begins around age 30, can be embraced (many great stylists love it!) or rejected. The good news is: there are solutions for everyone!

The first gray hair sounds the alarm, and it certainly won't be the last one you see! In fact, it all begins little by little around your hairline. Gray hair slowly takes over the rest of your head, signaling the decrease in progressive activity of the pigmentation cells, the melanocytes. This is an enzyme strike on your scalp, so to speak. Melanocytes are larger than the other cells, but they have the same lifespan.

CARING FOR GRAY HAIR Gray hair is gorgeous, pure refinement—as long as you prevent it from yellowing. Use iridescent shampoos and products that effectively prevent yellowing to preserve the subtle balance between salt and pepper. An ultra-stylish cut will create a striking look on a young face.

HIDING GRAY HAIR Tone-on-tone coloring will add subtleties to your color and cover grays so they fade into the rest of your hair. You can also style sections of your hair so the grays disappear.

Oxidation coloring is the best solution once you have more than 50 percent gray hair. Be sure to choose a color one or two shades lighter than your natural one. This method also has the benefit of softening your features.

If you pull a gray hair, it will grow back gray, and runs the risk of disrupting the hair cycle and losing that strand of hair for good.

ADVICE FROM COLORIST RODOLPHE
Gray hair is most obviously visible at the root. Along the shaft of the hair, it tends to blend in with the rest. This is why it is usually enough to color only the crown and allow the ends to do their own thing.

Six out of ten women color their hair, and among them, four in ten do it to cover gray.

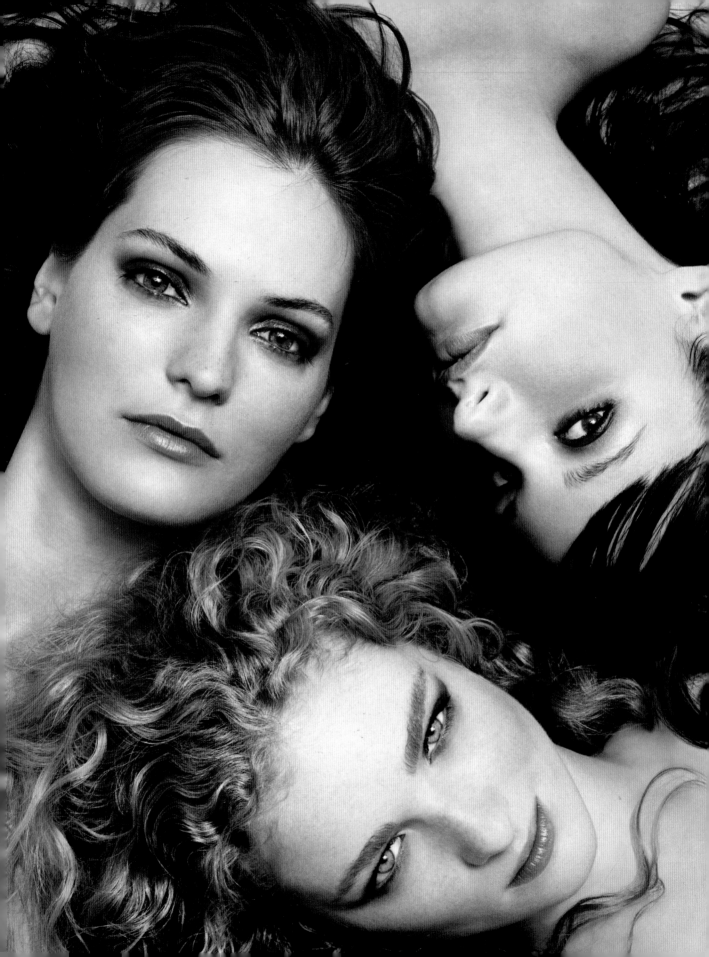

Rodolphe
Colorist

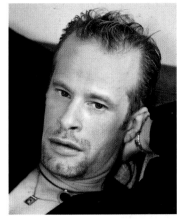

His paternal grandmother was a watercolorist, he owes his career to a painting by Cocteau, and he learned that the apartment where he set up his bedroom salon, "Color by Rodolphe," belonged to Picabia. It is difficult to imagine a more promising number of coincidences for giving women the color of their dreams.

"I played the role of pioneer… but women are the ones who invented the colorist!"

Perhaps being deaf since I was 10 years old has sharpened my eye. Marguerite, my paternal grandmother, was a watercolorist, and she was my first master. She explained to me that **objective color does not exist, each of us "fabricates" our own,** interpreting the light reflected on an object and then having the optic nerve transmit the information to the brain.

She guided my first steps, from watercolor, which is diluted into an immediate shading, to modeling clay, which makes art palpable by associating it with touch.

I DID NOT WANT TO BECOME A STYLIST; I ONLY WANTED TO DO COLOR.

When I first started out, however, the two jobs were combined, and people did not make a distinction. The colorist was like a sous-chef in a restaurant, and was simply there to hide a gray hair or transform a brunette into a platinum blonde. To prove yourself, you "did a color" behind a folding partition. It was a bit shameful—you applied it, set the timer, and rinsed. It was a no-brainer. ▶

The symbiosis of three emblematic images of femininity—blonde, red, and brunette—a canvas to encompass all the beauties of the world.

"When I first started out, you 'did a color' behind a folding partition only to hide gray hair. . . it was a bit shameful."

Only the great styling houses like Carita and Alexandre de Paris had their own colorists. I actually dreamed of working at Alexandre: When I arrived in Paris, I accepted a bunch of small jobs, but I wrote him a letter once a month for eleven months. With the eleventh negative response, the director finally granted me a meeting at Avenue Matignon, thanked me for my perseverance, and explained that they trained colorists there in the same way monks get their training in a monastery and that they had no need for me. As I was leaving, Alexandre saw me pass and hired me with these enigmatic words: "Jean would have really liked this one…"

He thought I looked like a painting by Cocteau, his friend who passed away years before. These little events have a touch of destiny about them.

I spent fifteen wonderful years with Alexandre: Between movie stars, queens, and empresses, I lived in a champagne bubble. But he taught me more than just my trade.

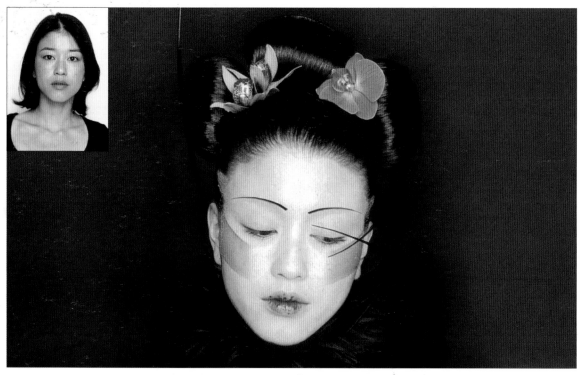

Three new takes on classic looks.
1. The impression of blonde bands and the chromatic blend creates a beautiful surprise with the addition of an orchid.

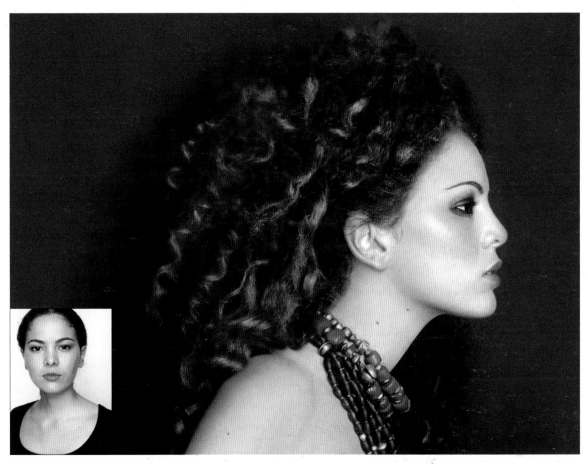

2. *Thick hair, sandy highlights—we used a product to remove color, mixed with oxidants and sand, to prevent uniform coloring and give hundreds of reflections. The result is a look that is very close to natural, one you get from being out in the sun, for example.*

He taught me how to look at women, to decode their language, to really listen to them. He gave me a true education in women.

I cannot thank him enough in one lifetime!

I have humbly tried to continue the spirit of his work. He brought me along, at the exact moment that the hair color trend exploded in the early '80s, when it had reached the street— just as he'd predicted it would. His motto, which he loved to repeat, was: "We create the trends on the third floor, and years later we find them on the street."

I became a pioneer of making color service part of the whole salon experience, and I quickly attained a high profile in the media. Thanks to a wave of American actresses who changed their hair color—like Meryl Streep and Cameron Diaz—the myth of Jean Harlow, Joan Crawford, and Marilyn Monroe was broken. The fairly easy bottle blonde that drove men wild was no longer the only color to have.

▶

"Women are the ones who invented colorists!"

Color spread like wildfire, and it was embraced everywhere. Women began to come in for nothing but color, and the colorist was finally recognized. This changed everything—it was a true revolution.

Women are the ones who invented colorists!

The feeling when you are about to color hair is identical to the one when you find yourself in front of a blank canvas with a paintbrush. What happens to the person's face is magical and profound.

My ideal of working at home did not happen until Juliette Gréco, a famouss French actress and singer, found me a place. It was then that "Color by Rodolphe" was born [1997]. Everything followed after that. My driving force was recklessness, and that helped me.

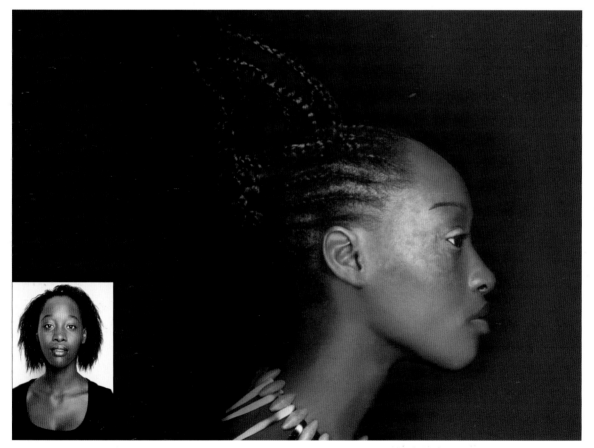

3. The blue reflections at the slightest change in position warm the skin to highlight this use of tone-on-tone.

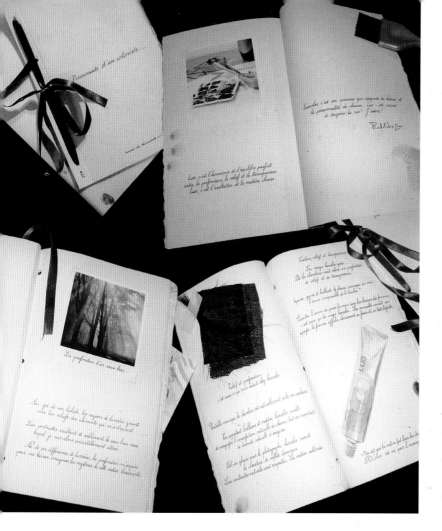

The most beautiful coincidence is that the painter Picabia, the master of color, lived in the apartment where I set up my studio! And he was a friend of my grandfather. Everything happened so quickly once I opened my "color apartment" (I never refer to it as a salon); the infatuation began immediately. There were more women than chairs when I opened! Many people helped me, it was fantastic. I even have photos of Juliette Gréco in the middle of a job.

HOW TO COLOR

A first visit takes place in an office since it's more intimate. This is where I get a general sense of the individual, man or woman.

I am very in touch with the person in front of me, it simply has to do with a mutual understanding, nothing indiscreet. I don't want to change them just for change's sake. Nor do I restrict their decision simply based on their complexion or clothing. It's a lesson in color, the sensation of a beautiful material, and we walk a fine line: we make the difference between the good and the spectacular! Of course, there are still certain people who request the exact same blonde as Madonna.

Hair is the last thing that I look at on a woman—I see her walk, her attitude, the way she holds her hands: The color of her hair has to be in sync with all of those. You have to be in the sensory world, after you place the restrictions and codes—social, professional, sexual, to determine her own specific codes—and then move towards color or noncolor! You can also just as easily suggest to a woman a variation of her own color, or tell her to change nothing—that she looks perfect just as she is.

Color is not stable; it evolves all the time. It is an instant, an attitude, a way of understanding and determining a person. It's amazing—there are no fixed rules.

THE CLASSES OF THE COLORIST

I offer master classes for colorists. I am inspired by everything, and I explain to them that color creates emotions, with Yves Klein Blue, the young girl in the turban by Vermeer, Botticelli's Venus. ▶

"Of course, some women come in only to ask me for Madonna's blonde!"

I tell them: "You are the artists, you create emotion with your paintbrush, you must not forget the woman in front of you. Break the routine that you have become accustomed to."

I help them to recognize the value of their actions. It is such an opportunity to participate in the creation of emotion! To emphasize what I'm saying, I suggest to them that they color with watercolors, on a white sheet of paper. My role is to modestly show them the impact of their actions on a woman. They must be aware of their art in order to be an artist!

Our vocabulary is limited—the word "blonde" is going to evoke a precise shade for an individual person, and each has their own! We speak two different languages: Women speak a language of emotion, and stylists have our jargon.

When a woman comes in saying, "I want to be a blonde or a redhead," you do not have the right to disappoint her with your lack of interest or attention, both of which are disrespectful. Many have saved for six months to be there. You must think about the woman who got up that morning only to go to your studio, which is often precisely the case.

Coloring has become an act of beauty, an entirely social act, a true act of great trust and humility—you allow someone to intervene in your image and your integrity. You place your hair in the hands of another: what proof of love and confidence!

You must forget qualifications to allow observation to take over, forget all the rules of coloring and styling hair and leave everything to imagination.

You will know if you don't have the right color. When a woman is not happy for any number of reasons, she must find herself again, alone in front of her mirror, without artifice. Color is fluid and changeable, and she must actively participate in it.

Python in your hair! *The color is striking and worth seeing even without a face. The color calls to mind the snake, which in the Far East is the symbol of beauty and femininity—perfectly illustrating the metamorphosis of color and movement. Its scales evoke those of hair, and at first glance you don't necessarily even notice the snake. You need 125 colors to get this shade of sandy blonde!*

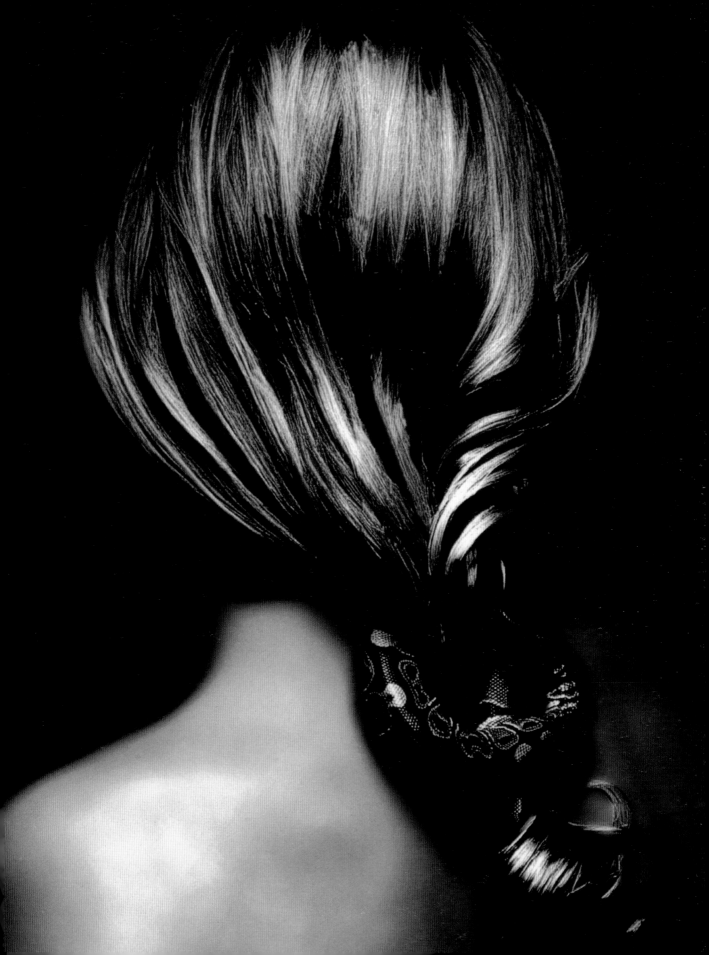

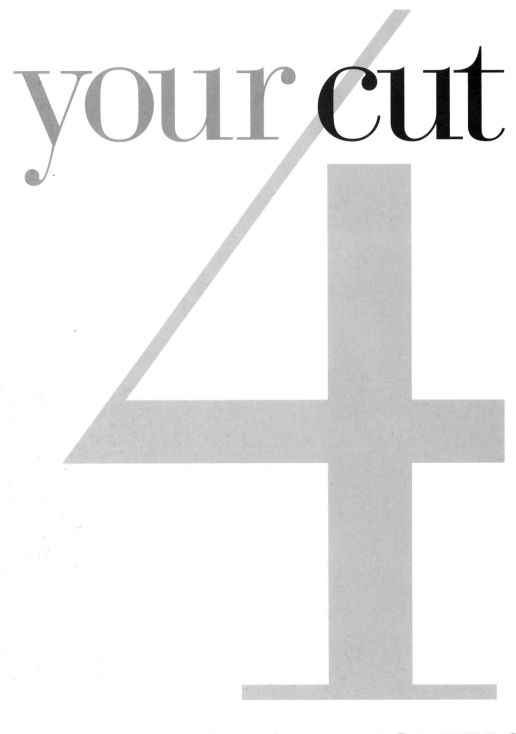

your cut

4

TECHNIQUES AND POINTERS

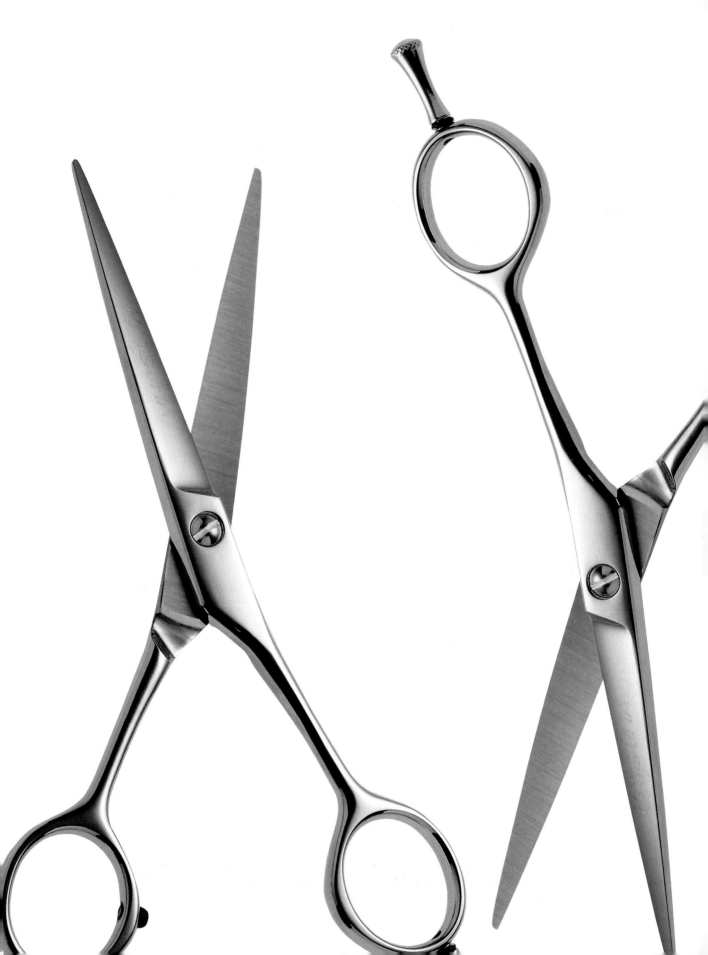

Change
revive
evolve
enhance
your
style...

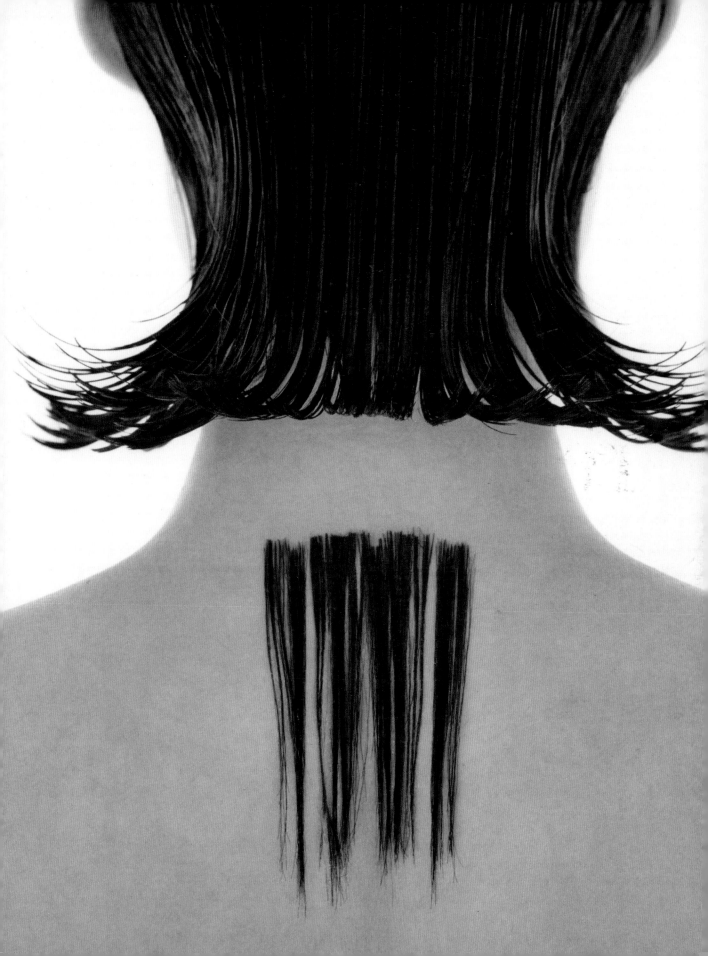

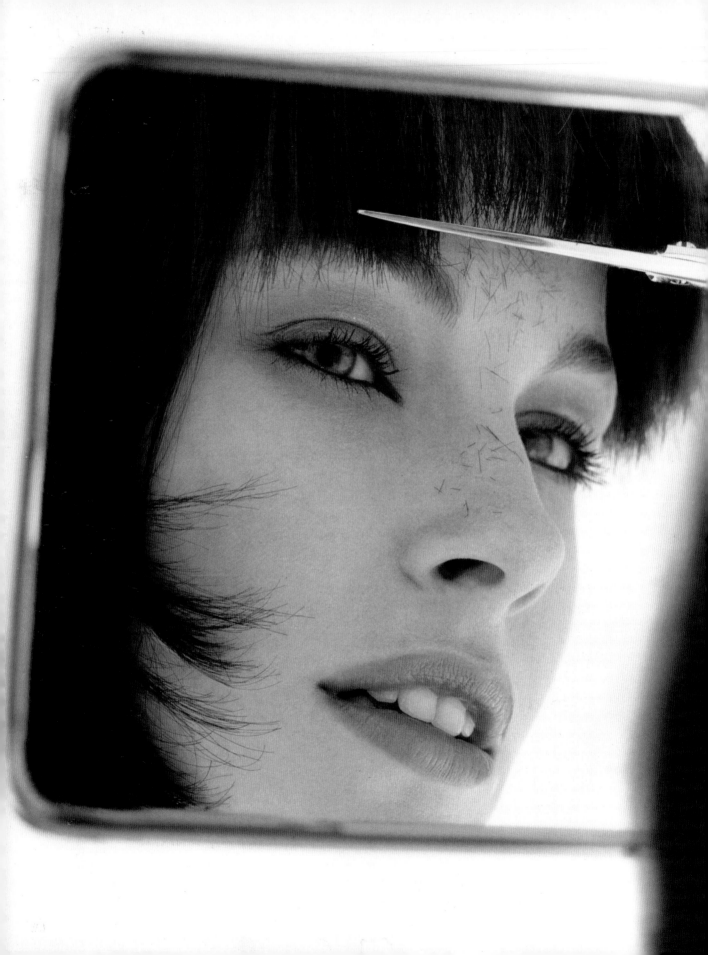

Cutting through the myths

How do you tell the true from the false? A quick review of good and bad habits to save your hair from common mistakes.

WANT TO CHANGE YOUR HAIRSTYLE? Don't do it on an impulse! **Talk with your stylist,** the best person to advise you, based not only on the shape of your face, but also your entire figure, the nature of your hair, and your lifestyle. And be sure to ask good questions and explain your motivation.

RESPECT THE NATURE OF YOUR HAIR. It is not impossible to dream outside your life: A fantasy hairstyle for one night is not a problem, but for everyday, choose a look that is suitable for your lifestyle.

CHANGE YOUR CUT = CHANGE YOUR COLOR? These are two inseparable issues that are essentially one! A color formulated to accentuate your face will put the finishing touches on a new cut by highlighting the layers, volume, and movement.

CUTTING YOUR HAIR MAKES IT THICKER? Of course not! A good cut is great for eliminating the ends (especially if they are split), but the nature of our hair is genetically programmed.

GO A THIRD OF AN INCH SHORTER WITH EACH BIRTHDAY? Put to rest the rule that says short hair is mandatory when you get older. The only trend that counts is doing what you want!

ADVICE FROM STYLIST JEAN-MARC MANIATIS
The best cut for you? There are computer programs that allow you to visualize yourself with countless different looks, but they do not take into account how your hair grows or the shape of your face. Trying on wigs doesn't help much either. The most reliable way is still simulating your future cut with clips at your salon.

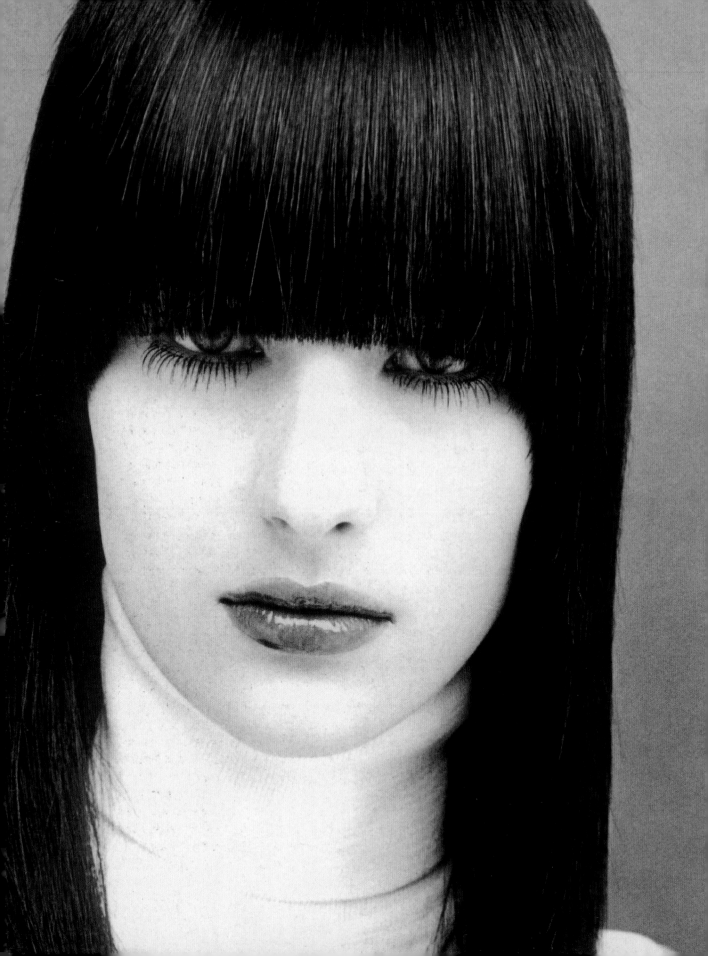

"I like my hair long"

How do you choose? Taking into account the shape of your face and your way of life, all cuts are permitted. One golden rule: Be yourself.

THE SEDUCTIVE APPEAL OF LONG HAIR corresponds to a type of woman who is glamorous without ever sacrificing her modernity. There is a tendency to really play up long hair as a **beauty accessory** in itself, placing it behind your ears or shading yourself behind it.

But neglecting it is not allowed: It is essential to give long hair shape and structure, cutting it at least once a season to freshen up the ends and bring back some volume. And you must avoid the overgrown teenager look, especially after age 45.

UPKEEP FOR LONG HAIR

Medium and long hair requires much more attention and constant care. This is why you should use **conditioners** on the ends only. Even if the rest of your hair is in good health, the ends are where you will have problems with tangling and dryness.

You can **leave your hair down** the day you shampoo, but put it up the next day. A loose braid or a soft chignon works well as long as you leave it alone. No touching!

At-home **coloring** is not recommended because long hair is more fragile and more difficult to work with than short hair.

ADVICE FROM HAIR RESEARCHER JEAN-MICHEL STURLA

WHY DOES HAIR GET MORE DAMAGED AT THE ENDS?
If you look at long hair under a microscope, it will be intact near the roots but will show signs of age (raised scales, split ends) the further down you go. The ends are the most damaged, but are also the "oldest." With hair growing about a third of an inch per month, if you have shoulder-length hair (about eight inches long), your ends will have already seen about twenty months of blowdrying, washing, coloring, and exposure. So even though hair is "dead," it still has a life!

"I like my hair short"

What's the benefit of short hair? Here is a rundown of all the arguments to keep in mind before making the jump.

SHORT STORY Short hair is ideal for accentuating an oval face or a long neck, for highlighting your face and affirming your personality, often giving the impression of a pixie. It also has the benefit of being easy to maintain as long as you begin with a good base: an impeccable cut.

And for that, **a stylist you trust is essential.** He or she must not only know your tastes before finding a style that works in harmony with your identity, but also the way your hair is going to react and naturally fall into place—especially when you go home to style it yourself!

GOING SHORT SAFELY

With a round face, you can do almost anything—including feathered layers. If your hair is a bit flat, you need to add volume, and if it's fine, it's better to keep a bit of extra length. **A long neck** looks great bare. **Large shoulders** will appear even larger with short hair: If this is your worry, avoid having hair cut straight across the nape. If you have a **pear-shaped figure,** it would be best to avoid a pixie cut; choose a square bob instead.

Reveal your ears? This is a great way to brighten your face!

With fine hair, layering at ear level will give you volume. **Thick hair** needs a good, clean cut with scissors.

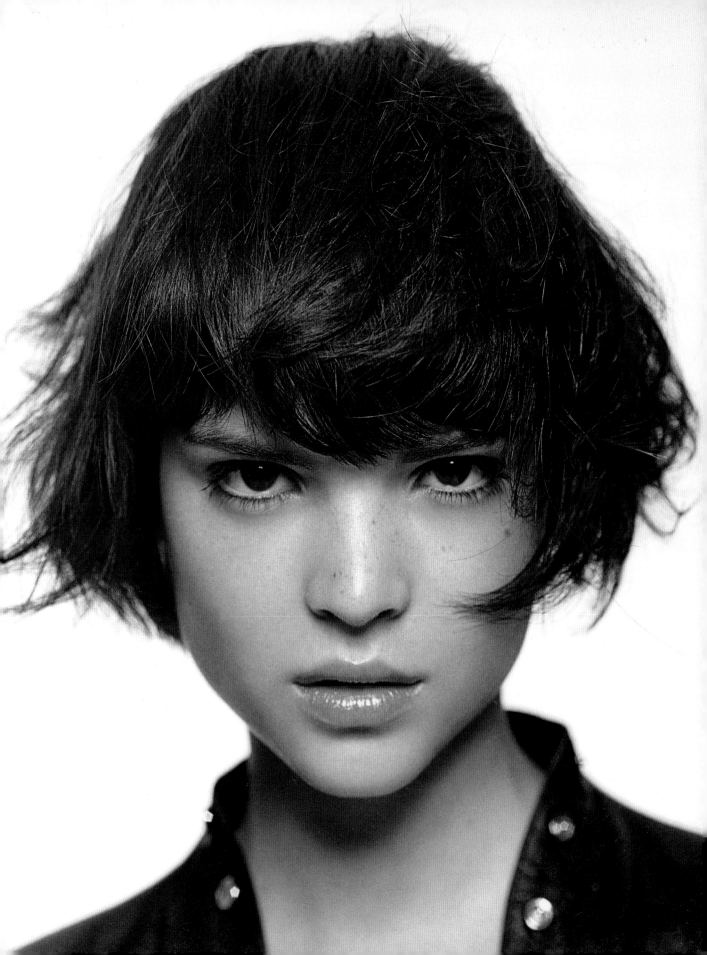

Quick tips from a pro

The unbelievable dexterity of a master with scissors, in a brilliant demonstration of the always fashionable pixie cut.

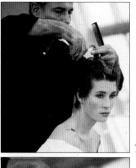

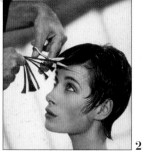

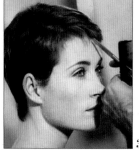

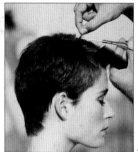

FOREVER SHORT!

1 PLAY WITH COLOR On such a small sur-face, anything goes. You can reinforce your natural color by darkening it (this page), or go with a complete contrast (far right).

2 EXPERT SNIPPING Ceramic scissors are used to transform any little defects in hair growth into aesthetic trump cards.

3 SMART LAYERS So that a short cut does not become too severe, you must know how to play with volume and bring softness to the lines.

4 PHENOMENAL WAVES Understanding how to work with them is critical to perfecting the design. "They bring life to a haircut, but you must know how to use them to your advantage."

5 IRRESISTIBLE RESULTS Ultra-feminine and face-highlighting, this style is very easy to maintain.

ADVICE FROM STYLIST JEAN-MARC MANIATIS
A men's haircut looks great on women with fine features, but its androgynous look also contrasts nicely with a feminine style.

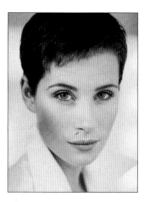

The result above is reinterpreted in platinum at right.

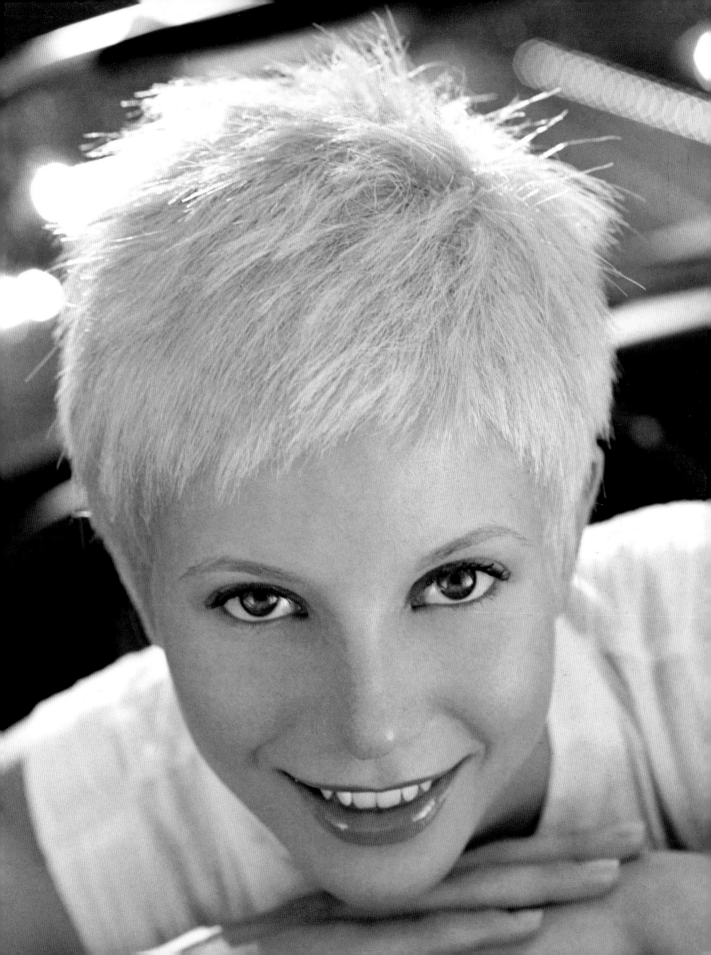

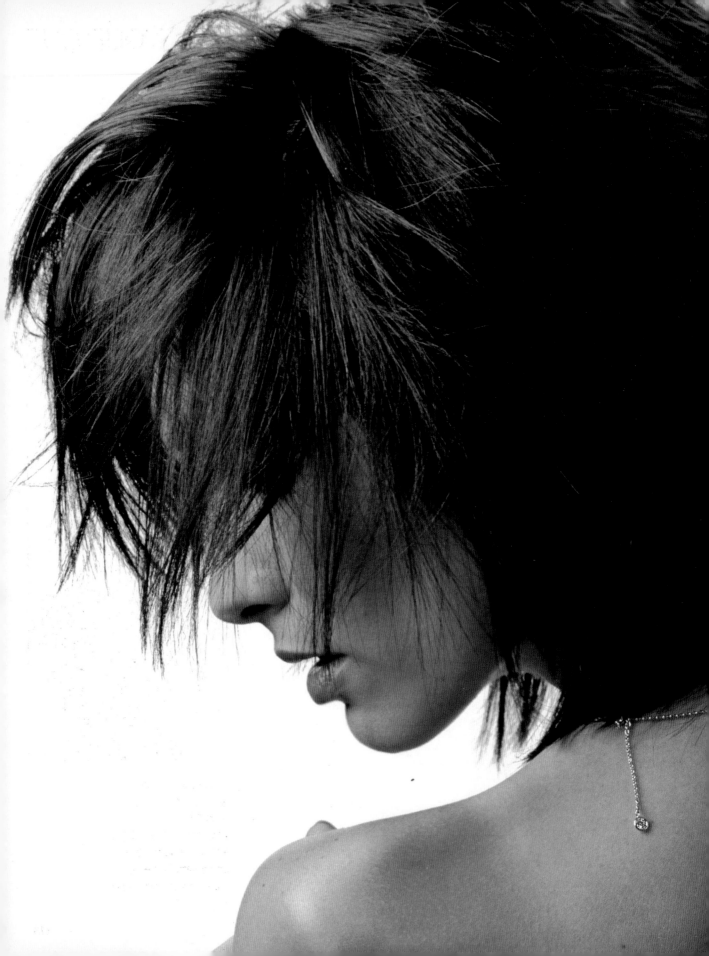

Perfect cuts for looking younger

The right hairstyle has the allure, the body, and the elegance to help keep your true age a secret!

COVER your neck and allow a few pretty pieces to caress it. Your neck is where the first signs of aging appear, even when your face is still supple.

Keeping your hair a bit longer at your nape with an asymmetrical bang is another winning strategy.

LAYERS will give the effect of lightness, while a severe hairstyle will certainly make you look older. To turn back time, wage war against flat hair and add layers at the crown.

Stylist John Nollet uses tricks of light to his client's advantage, sculpting locks of hair forward on the jawline to give the immediate impression of appearing ten years younger and five pounds lighter.

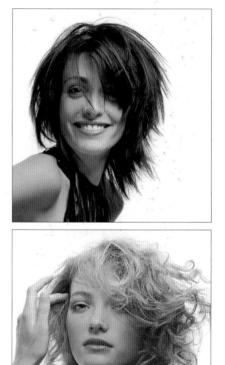

ADVICE FROM STYLIST JOHN NOLLET
Take advantage of light and movement—the immediate lift will give you pep and brightness.

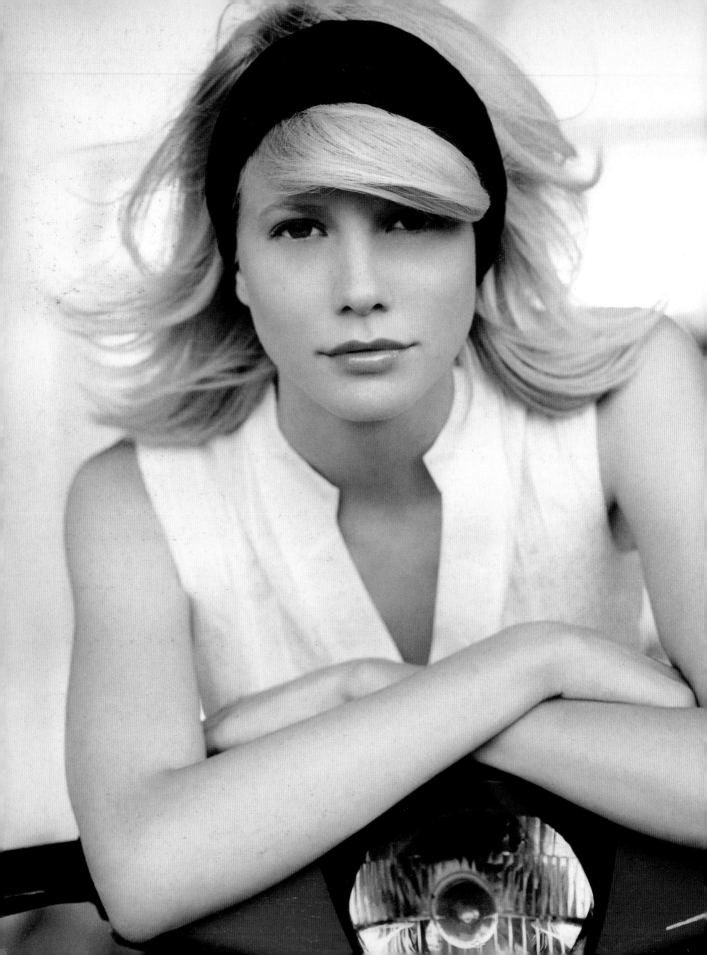

Jean-Marc Maniatis

Avant-Garde Stylist

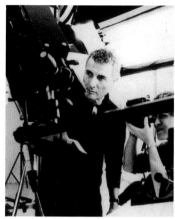

He started a revolution in the '70s by doing away with dowdy haircuts and creating wild and rebellious styles. Making women sexy while still giving them their freedom is the double credo of this eternally youthful man who continues to style hair ahead of his time.

> "If I invented a **cut** and it was not **immediately copied,** I did not force it— it's the person on the street **who decides.**"

I was 13 years old when it hit me. My cousin, a stylist in a large salon, asked me if I wanted to go to the movies with him, so I went to the reception area to wait. I was immersed in the distinctive, unmistakable smells of the salon—and then there were the women, each one more beautiful than the last. Two hours of waiting and it was over—I was seduced!

The stylists in the '60s had much more power over women, who came to have their hair done twice a week at least.

YOU DID NOT DO YOUR OWN HAIR, structural cuts did not exist, and the stylist's master touch was indispensable.

When I got back home, everyone thought it was a passing fancy at first, but in the end my father enrolled me in stylist's school. But I got the feeling I was wasting my time there. I found it too traditional, that it was not the thing for me. I was attracted by style and fashion magazines. Three years of school? No way! I took the shortcut.

I went to a great Greek stylist on Avenue Montaigne, but that was not a good fit for me either. He introduced me to stylist Jacques Dessange, and I became his assistant. It was my first studio session with a famous photographer and a very well-known model, and I was really impressed. It was in Orly, in a model of the Caravelle—he was the first to do fashion photos there. What an initiation! ▶

"The absence of **restrictions**, the **simple** act of allowing hair to dry **naturally**, that was truly a **revolution!**"

I went from photo shoot to photo shoot with Dessange, then moved to Carita during their great period. Everything happened so quickly. I had talent, but I did not realize I was still a beginner. At home, I was immersed. My father was a great Parisian boot maker, the equivalent of a famous fashion designer. He made shoes for Chanel and the models in her collections. My mother had a great sense of style. One day, she let me cut her hair and said, "You have made me look so young!" At that moment, I realized I was not meant to style but to embellish. It was instinctive.

Little by little, I began to cut hair within a very select group. The tennis champion Grinda entrusted me with her long hair when I was only 16, if you can believe it. The Carita sisters sent me to the theater to style hair for the stars of the era—from hairpieces for Ludmilla Tchérina to Bernard Blier. They sent me to Pierre Cardin as well, for the haute couture fashion shows. All these names that I once dreamed about were now people I actually knew.

I left Carita because I fell in love with the work of a great stylist, Thérèse Chardin, who refined and perfected the "feathered" look. She took me on in a heartbeat, and I stayed with her for two years. Then my father helped me open my first salon, Elrhodes, with my cousin on Avenue Mozart. I was 20 years old. We immediately got off to a good start. Dany Saval became a patron, and then Mylène Demongeot, Sophie Daumier, even Catherine Deneuve. We had models, actresses, and pop singers.

I also "created" the first Mireille Mathieu, the Pop Art version!

Then I moved on to Faubourg Saint-Honoré, franchises, Japan, before my cousin and I decided to go our separate ways—we had different aspirations. I took a break. I'd loved the spontaneity and creativity of those early years, and it wasn't fun and crazy anymore. I began again as a studio stylist. Peter Knapp and Hélène Lazareff asked me to become the stylist for their magazine—with the status of a journalist. I was present at all their meetings. A unique four-year experience—fashion, beauty—before launching my brand Maniatis in 1971. This was a true campaign—with magazines, of course. It was a journey that was helped along greatly by luck.

I was a perfectionist! I preferred not to expand my business, but rather, put my heart and soul into it personally.

▶

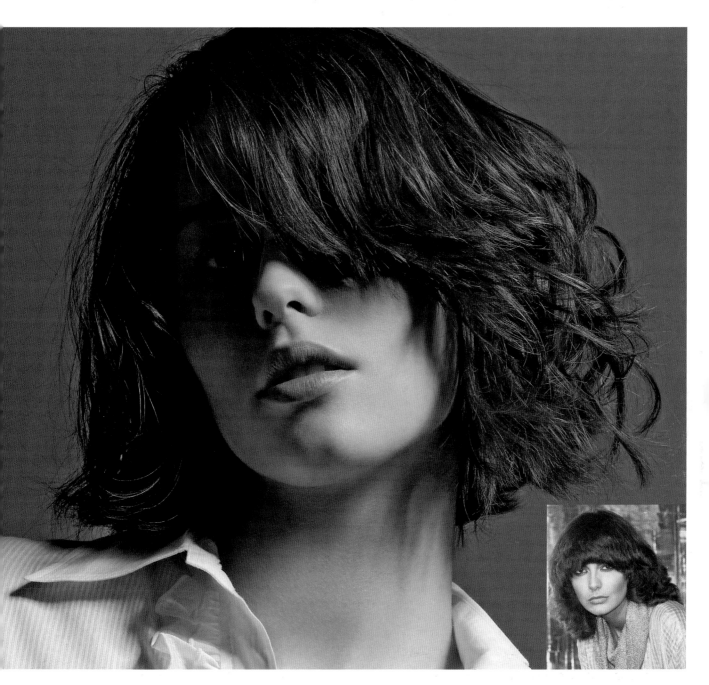

WILD WAVES, VINTAGE 1977 VERSION (inset, right) AND TODAY, 2007 (above)—
A Rolling Stones fan, I was fascinated by Mick Jagger's wild look, and I had to adapt it. I fine-tuned this technique, which I called "Sauvage" in honor of the film starring Catherine Deneuve. This was my first worldwide success. The name "the sauvage" cut was exported all the way to Japan, and like blue jeans, it went all around the world. It was sexy, it was feminine, it was adapted for every length. The contemporary version has much more pep, and the brunette color has reflections of Coca-Cola!

I HAVE ALWAYS HAD TWO ABSOLUTE RULES:

NUMBER 1: Make a woman attractive and sexy, which sparks desire. (How would I style her hair if I were going out with her that night?)

NUMBER 2: I believe in the principle of "let it go" if a style or cut is not copied right away. You cannot force it—it's up to the people on the street to decide.

MY LIFE… IN CUTS!

• **The pixie cut** 1969-1970 (see below) I did this style for two stars with very long hair who only worked with the Bourdins or the Newtons—Birgit and Suzanne—who were very feminine, not at all tomboys, with delicate features and fine hair. They had medium ashy hair, not very light, and on both of them I lightened around the face and all the edges. That changed everything, brightening and adding color at precise places. It was all a question of chance.

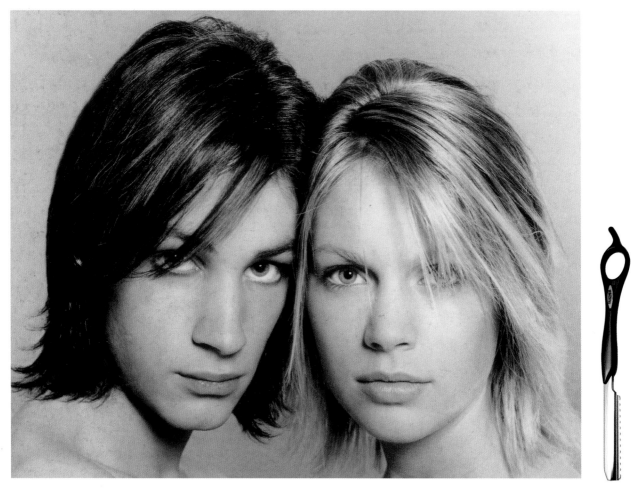

A magical tool that "feathers" hair,
to celebrate androgynous beauty.

• **The sauvage** (see page 117) You cannot patent a haircut, and all the women in the world did not come to me personally for it, but it was truly a revolution. Before this, cutting hair upside down was unthinkable. In school, I would have gotten a zero.

• **The first layered style** Long layers happened by accident (the word "layered" did not exist in this sense before). I was doing photo shoots with Helmut Newton in Deauville, and the model came in with very long hair in a bob. There was quite a bit of wind, but it did not blow the way we wanted, and her hair did not move well—it was plastered down. I began by pulling her hair up, but nothing was working. Finally, when two or three little sections came loose, all of a sudden I had an idea (not a stylist's idea, a photographer's idea): I cut a few more sections, and it was instantly graceful!

Two years later everything fell into place: I started working with hair from the crown to the ends, layering for lightness. This cut was contrary to all the rules: You usually start at the bottom! But my new method resulted in lots of volume and launched a trend. I produced this style at the same time as Dessange (with Bruno) and at Jean-Louis David, where sophisticated women became more liberated right away.

Young women did not want to look like their mothers, and my cuts were different. They met women's expectations because they had no restrictions: You were allowed to air-dry your hair—this was a true revolution!

IN THE SAME WAY THAT WOMEN WERE FREED FROM THE CORSET, I FREED THEM FROM THE SHACKLES OF THEIR MOTHER'S HAIRDRESSER!

• **The androgynous cut:** The world of Calvin Klein in New York inspired me to create a unique cut with this blade (photo at left), which, unlike a razor, does not remove volume from hair. This is the ideal tool to use for keeping hair very close to the head. It is somewhat difficult to master (you have the impression that you no longer have hair!), but a year later the technique took off. And it's still popular, seven years later, as one of the cuts that works great for almost everyone. It's basically the equivalent of jeans for hair!

It does not work for very curly hair (at least the naturally curly kind) except for one evening only.

The bob that works best is the one that has some movement and does not look too severe.

▶

"I wanted to stir things up in the field of color."

I spent my time inventing new techniques for very light blondes, using cosmetic colors: vivid but still pretty—blues and reds. Or you can dye a section of hair on each side of the part, creating a veil of color that blends into the rest of the hair and requires almost no maintenance.

In terms of highlights, if you apply the product after back-combing or teasing, you avoid roots and you only have to retouch three times a year rather than once a month!

As for the color "blue jean," I was fortunate to create it at the same time that Chanel was creating its makeup with faded shades, and combining the two produced a very Andy Warhol look.

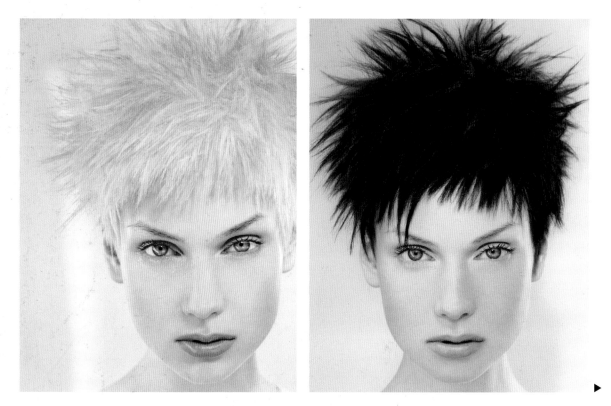

FADED BLUE JEAN *(far right) and two interpretations on the poles (above): glacier blue blonde for the North Pole and black with delicate blue reflections for the South Pole.*

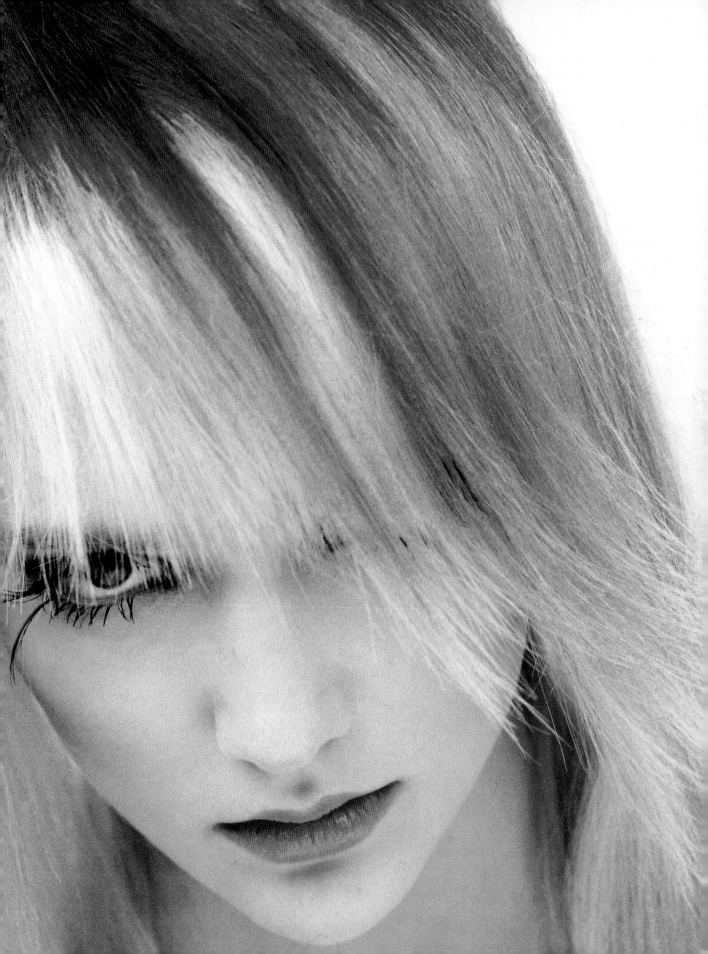

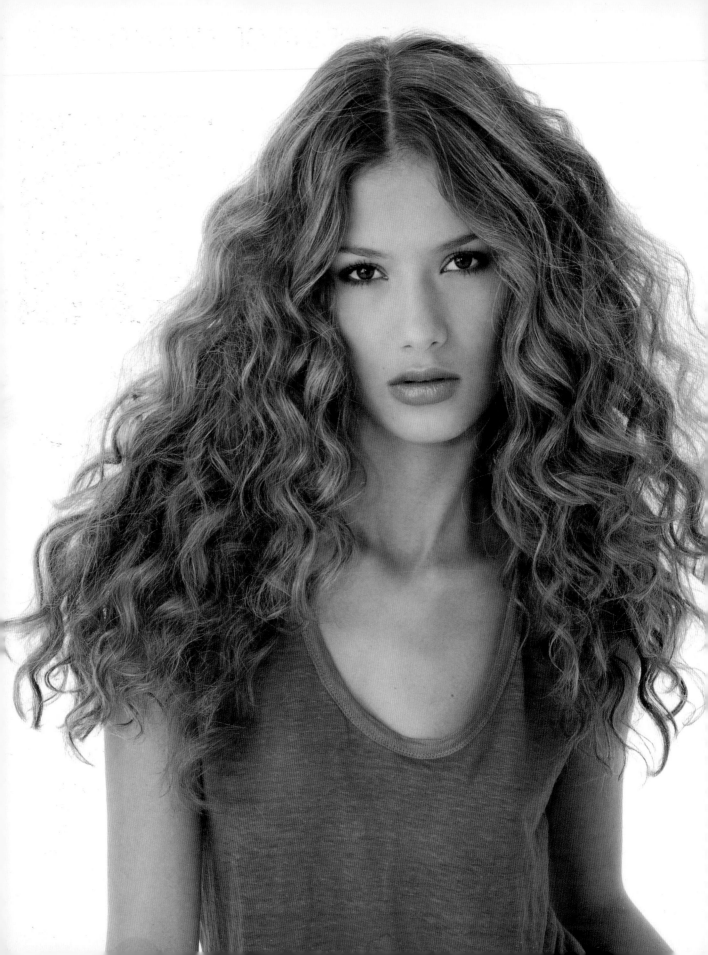

Éric Pfalzgraf

Designer Stylist

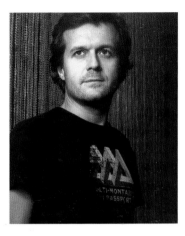

From his salon in the heart of Saint-Germain-des-Prés to Japan, from the beaches of St. Tropez to retreat spas and even prisons, no terrain is foreign to this visionary stylist, who has used his taste for beautiful work to passionately defend women's rights.

> "Fashion must be **at the service** of beauty: Beautiful skin and pretty hair, are the most **important things!**"

To be a stylist is one of the rare professions where you focus on the little girl hidden inside every woman, the one you want to find and protect.

There are endless surprises, protocol goes out the window, and intimacy takes over—notoriety does not come into consideration in these relationships.

Just as in a couple, your relationship with your stylist is challenged at every visit. The connection with a stylist depends upon how well he or she meets your demand for attention. There is an expectation.

A GOOD STYLIST IS ONE WHO OPENS TO A WOMAN A WHOLE WORLD OF POSSIBILITIES—AND ALLOWS HER TO EXPRESS HER FULL POTENTIAL IN A SALON VISIT.

You must allow the time and the means to combine all the elements needed to properly care for a woman. If she takes the initiative to come to you, it's not to get the same result she gets at home!

I did not choose this profession for the money or for the social status. I chose it based on only one consideration: what would my everyday routine look like? My father chose to be a chef, but I prefer the company of women to casseroles. I always wanted to be a bit different, a bit visionary, and to style the prettiest women in the world!

▶

The absolute beauty of outrageous curls . . .

"Being a stylist is a meeting with yourself. It can even sometimes give you back your reason to live."

I chose to practice my trade outside of salons, from the private beaches of St. Tropez to prisons, from hospitals to spa retreats—an itinerant salon, a meeting with self, with life, that's what's important. I worked at La Maison de Solenn, an adolescent health retreat in Paris, to offer young girls with eating disorders a reason to live again. They were ready to start eating healthily, to have beautiful hair, and I was able to teach them. I prefer to define my profession as one that works to make every day more beautiful. It's more useful than saying to myself that I am going to spend my life cutting hair that will just grow back again. I am still pushing my limits with regard to my love of the image: I take photos, I direct films, and I produce them as well (Célibataires).

GIFT, TALENT, OR WORK—WHAT COULD BE BETTER THAN PARTICIPATING IN REVEALING THE BEAUTY OF WOMEN? WHAT COULD BE BETTER?

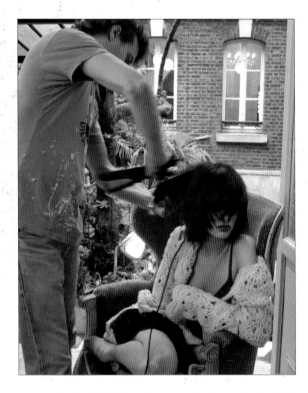

Indeed, this profession has lagged behind that of fashion designers or great chefs for a long time: Alain Ducasse and his team inspired me more than my peers. You cannot be on different wavelengths; the décor must be top notch. I opened my salon at Rue du Four, 11,000 square feet in the heart of the artist's quarter, and it was a true turning point for me. A jury came and decided, without my soliciting them at all, that it was the most beautiful salon in the world.

For me, beauty is number one, and fashion remains an accessory. Beautiful skin, pretty hair—these are the most important things.

Through my training and work with great product lines, I've found that beauty has become so powerful—we are dedicating more and more time to it and to our well-being. But today, our true rival is time (lunch, a trip to the gym). A trip to the salon is fun, like an impulse buy. ▶

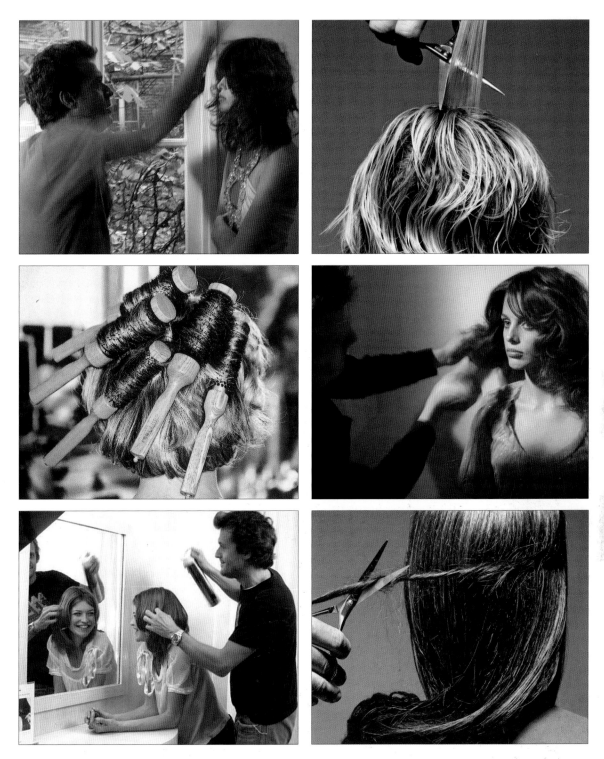

FEATS OF THE SALON *I never use a razor, always scissors—the stylist's perfect tool. THE PICKETING TECHNIQUE (top) is done exclusively with scissors to encourage volume. It will give texture and create thickness in fine hair. We avoid straight lines, and cutting ends at different lengths will prevent weightiness and create movement and softness. Hair will fall into place naturally. BACK-COMBING AND TEASING WITH SCISSORS or WINDING (bottom) will accentuate and create intentional imperfections, emphasizing the rebellious nature of hair. HAIRSPRAY will help define your style, but brush again to avoid the helmet effect!*

"Good taste does not exist as an absolute, but beautiful materials and natural glamour do."

When you go out for dinner, however sublime (I speak from experience, having taken over the family restaurant in Strasbourg), you enjoy your meal, leave, and then it's done. However, when you head home after a visit to your stylist, the result stays with you!

Sometimes we are "unstylists." A woman can come in very polished and leave a bombshell!

We want to make people happy: everyone is searching for perfection. The connection to beauty is unique. It's not about comparing yourself to the models on the glossy pages.

Good taste does not exist as an absolute, but natural glamour and beautiful materials do. A beautiful cut, where you know that the stylist has made you happy, is less beautiful than a pretty

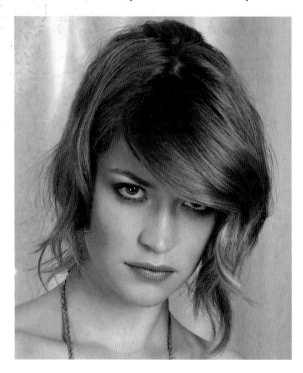

figure—so we're led to believe. But you must purge yourself of the negatives that you can learn in this profession.

The simplest things are often the best. The strange truth is, models always have the simplest hairstyles. I maintain that the 200 of us stylists do this look without "learning" it, a simple vintage "polish" with natural colors, and beautiful hair that emphasizes the style, not the opposite. With a thousand clients per day, you maintain hair. A great stylist does very little cutting, and clients come in only about once a year for a spectacular before-and-after. Otherwise, not much changes, which is perhaps a very good thing for the stylist.

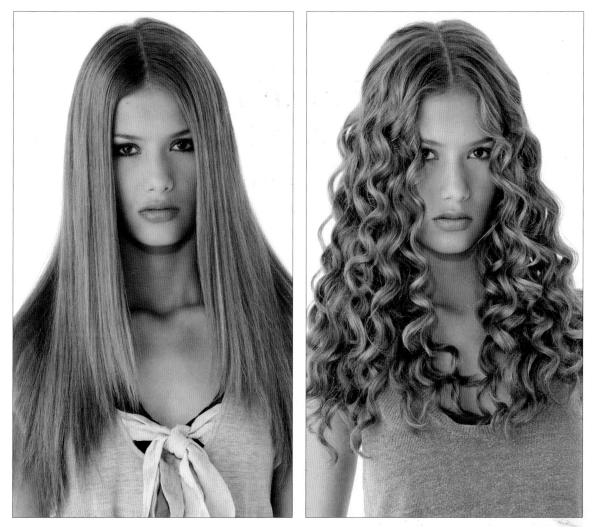

FROM SLEEK AND STRAIGHT *Hair is styled section by section with a flatiron for reflective shine. For simple styling, flip your head over and blow-dry, alternating warm air (for volume) and cool air (to make hair shiny).*

. . . ***TO DEFINED CURLS*** *Wind hair around a spiral curling iron for perfect definition. Another option is updated pin curls, using thermal brushes as rollers to create natural waves (see page 125).*

HANDBOOK OF OUR SECRETS

I find it rewarding that our clients can figure out the key techniques of our profession.

We conduct tests to determine the state of the scalp and the hair itself, which can be brittle, dried out, soft, or solid—to better determine which products to use.

WE DO NOT CUT, WE REDESIGN All our cuts add body to hair, and that means something to women! When a woman comes to see us, she has expectations. Women don't want to put up with their flaws; they come in hoping for results. But the client must express her wishes! ▶

"Sometimes we are 'unstylists.' A woman can come in very polished and leave a bombshell!"

Our style is mainly natural, shoulder-length hair. We create imperfections with scissoring techniques, making hair more natural than natural itself! We are looking for glamour, not for excessive sexiness. We aim for vintage natural; I do not try to be trendy. This style is very Saint-Germain-des-Prés and was exported to Japan. The result is the most beautiful hair possible with a pretty shape and style. We work with hair in such a way that when it grows back in, it does so in the best way.

COLORING We use the existing base color, analyze it, and begin with the most obvious thing: that the eye is accustomed to your color. Today, the truly natural seems boring to us. We need to enhance it, but with discretion.

I add a drop of olive oil to my color treatments to protect the scalp and to slightly reduce the absorption and give color more transparency—my Italian roots are never far away!

Get rid of highlights; long live the polish of natural color! The polishing technique is done with a paintbrush, and it will enhance the effects of the cut, with V-shaped sections and the new growth in layers, to create contrasts. Polishing gives the effect of volume, but not monochromatic hair.

STYLING, STRAIGHTENING, AND DRYING do not ruin hair. This becomes obvious when you consider that models are styled ten times a day and still have beautiful hair.

Perms are recommended on a case-by-case basis, but they are very rare today and are practically only done on Japanese women!

Hairspray? Yes, and we even use of one of L'Oréal's vintage varieties. I love the smell—my grandmother used it! Don't use it to stiffen your hair, though. If your hair is too clean, you will not be able to create styles. Use hairspray to better define the style. To avoid the helmet effect, brush your hair out again after spraying.

Teasing and back-combing? Yes, for a fashion show, but not for every day!

MISTAKES TO AVOID Cuts that are too short, even when there is volume, and on the flip side, hair that is too long when there is no volume. And too much lightener or peroxide.

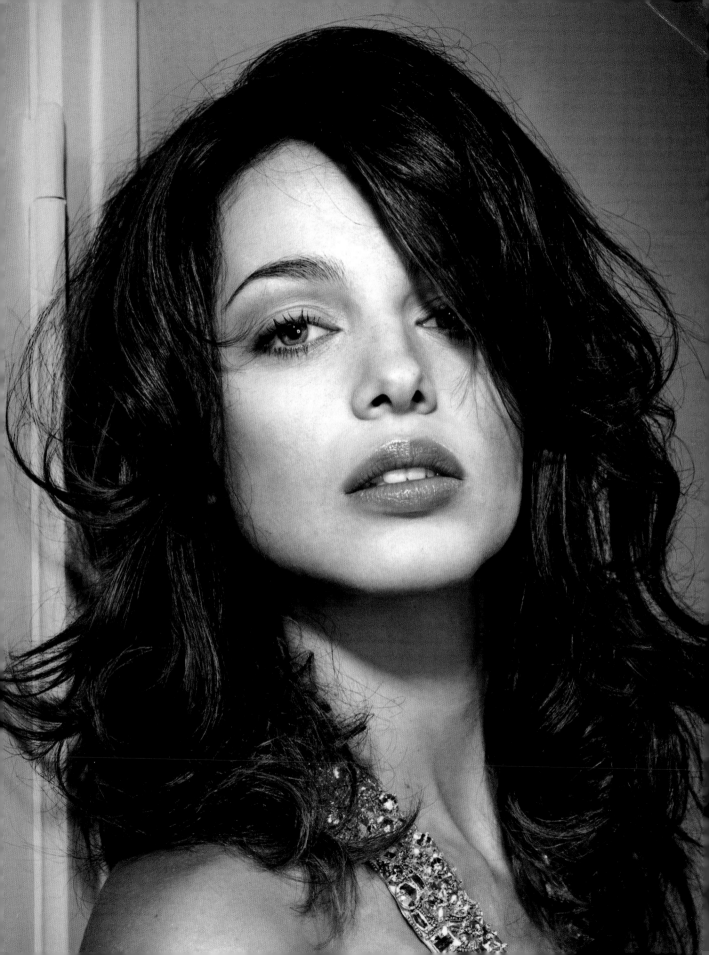

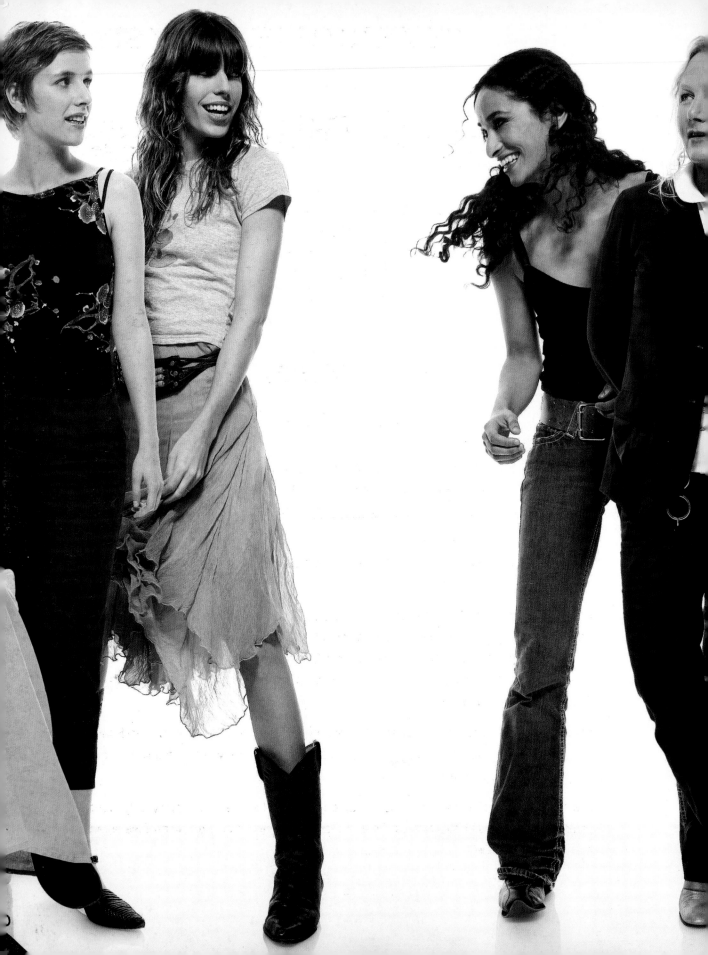

Bernard Friboulet

Stylist

Très Confidentiel, an intimate space like a theater dressing room, radiates with the personality of this gifted man who styles celebrities like Sharon Stone but who will also go to the ends of the earth to help women take matters into their own hands.

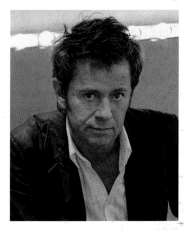

"It's all a matter of feeling. Psychology is truly 50 percent of our profession."

To speak of a luxury stylist today means nothing. We should remain humble. I never feel superior to the person who is sitting in front of me. Just because you have tools in your hand doesn't mean you don't have to respect another person. Respect is the foundation of every relationship.

Expectations have evolved. A woman wants to be beautiful, have her own cut, feel good, and be able to style her hair easily.

I called my salon Très Confidentiel to pique curiosity, to intrigue people, and make them wonder what they might find behind the curtains. It's not that the salon is not open to everyone, but I created it with a particular image in mind. It's very white, very Zen, very pure. The decoration does not take over; it's the functional destination that takes precedence—with the spirit of a theater dressing room.

I started my vocational training at age 14, had my first salon at 24, and moved to Paris at 30. Then I met Jean-Claude Gallon, which opened to doors to the world of fashion and cinema and helped me to evolve.

I was the leader of a team of fifteen people in Rue St-Honoré, but I really only wanted to practice my trade as I had always dreamed, devoting my self only to my profession and not managing personnel.

▶

"I can't do two things, at once — it would be like painting two identical canvases."

Today I have only two assistants, we work by appointment only, and never have more than two clients at a time. This builds loyalty and encourages meaningful moments. These moments are sacred, focused exclusively on the client, unlike the hustle and bustle of a jam-packed salon. I love the way I practice my trade and don't get bored with it.

I have never forced ideas—they come on their own, when they are ready.

Even my prices are not out of reach. I have many clients who travel from other countries and who are happy to come to me every three months! A satisfied women will return, but she doesn't need to do so more than every two or three months—her color will hold, and she has better things to do than go to the stylist every week. She would much rather have fun.

With our new way of life, there is not one particular day of the week when you have to be better styled than any other. You wash your hair every day because pollution requires it. Your hairstyle has become an accessory, just like pumps or a handbag, and a cut needs to be changeable throughout the day, from very sporty to more sophisticated.

There are no fixed trends, all textures and all cuts are permitted.

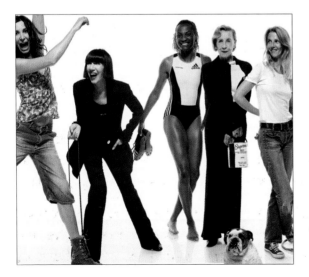

MY APPROACH TO COACHING
My clients so often say to me "Yes, but what happens when I get home?" So I arrange three-hour meetings with them to teach them how to do their own hair.

I start my training session with choosing the right shampoo and styling products. Then we talk about how to hold the dryer, direct its heat, and, if necessary, use a brush as you dry. I then demonstrate how to make a chignon without the claw clasps that I detest, and how to make a ponytail at the correct height.

I also show how to trim your bangs with manicure scissors to avoid catastrophes (it requires two people).

I work on the entire personality of a woman, on her way of being and moving, not simply on her face. If you don't know how to analyze the woman in front of you within a few seconds, you need to change professions!

Stylists receive classical training in cutting and styling, but once these essentials are acquired, it's up to you to be creative. They don't teach you psychology even though it's 50 percent of the job.

You must adapt because each woman dreams of something different, even if she pretends not to have specific wishes.

You must find the right words, the ones that will help release the expression of her desires, put you in connection with her, like in the theater: everything is a matter of feeling.

Ideas come immediately; this is an instinctual profession. Generally, women will open up very quickly, and the dialogue will start right away.

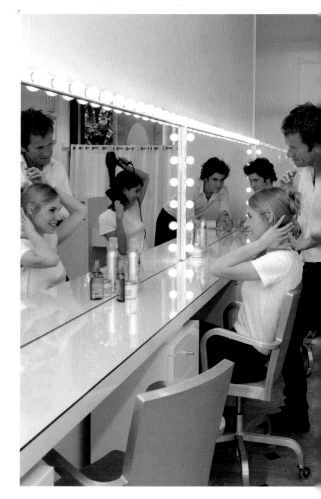

MY MUSES

Although they are actresses by profession, they are all still simply women.

Take for example **Sophie Marceau.** She is as natural when she comes into my salon as any of my other clients.

I never let myself go overboard, even with Sharon Stone. Nonetheless, with her, I was a bit nervous at first. And then, the moment I began preparing her color and took the brush in my hand, the magic of the trade brought down all the barriers, and I was able to see her as I see all of my clients.

With actress Gong Li, trust came very gradually. The first time that I put her hair up, I gave her the hairpins and she put them in. And then little by little, she let me do it. I even managed to give her bangs, even though she never wore them before. Everything can happen with respect, once trust is won. ▶

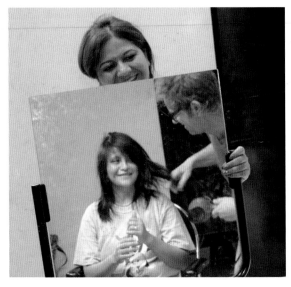
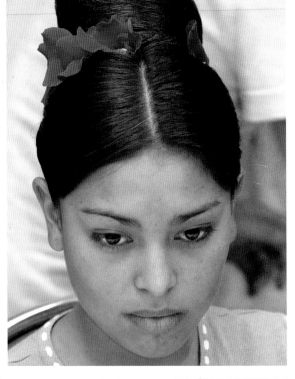
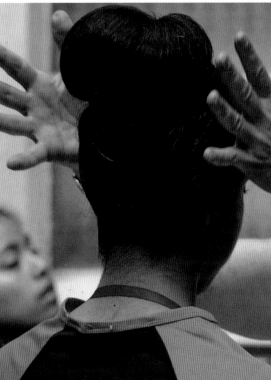
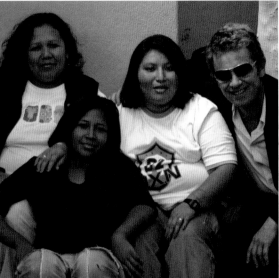

HELPING WOMEN BOOST THEIR CONFIDENCE?
I AM VERY PROUD OF IT. . . BUT DON'T MISTAKE ME
FOR THE HOLY FATHER OF STYLISTS!

L'Oréal accompanied me on a journey that I hold very dear to my heart: Hairstyling for everyone! *in Guatemala where I joined with the organization* Three Quarters of the World, *in the headquarters of* Solo Para Mujeres *(Just for Women), for our first mission in November 2006 (which they conducted again in 2007). The goal? To give women the great job security to train them to become stylists, but more importantly to give them back their pride and desire to be beautiful. Frédéric Bazin, who is an actor, worked with them on their walk and demeanor. It also had the benefit of putting ideas in place: You must never forget your roots.*

"If you don't know how to **analyze** the woman in **front of you** within a few seconds, you need to **change** professions!"

Any time I start feeling apprehensive, my passion for the profession makes it disappear, and that's such a powerful thing. What I respect above everything else is elegance. In every circumstance. Self-respect and elegance of the heart are far more important that physical appearances.

Elegance is a pair of shoes, a handbag. Or a haircut, which you hope looks elegant when you run into a woman who is a client of yours.

I have also worked on films—for Agnès Jaoui, I created all the styles for *La Maison de Nina*—but the life of a stage stylist is not for me. Even if Gong Li and Aishwarya Rai asked for me, I could not be away on tour for two months.

I worked with great creative minds like Issey Mikayé, and did research on different cultures. This is a profession that allows you to explore the universe.

I needed a place to land, somewhere that allowed me to remain grounded in reality. I work just four days a week, then the rest of the time I recharge my batteries. The street inspires me, the terraces and the bistros, an expo, everything awakens my curiosity. I adore taking the metro.

A WOMAN WOULD NEVER DARE ENTER A SALON SIMPLY TO REQUEST A CONSULT.
I invented "advice days" during which I do twenty-minute consultations, far too short a time to actually style hair. These are intended for women who want to make a change but not necessarily make an appointment with me. After their consult, they can just as easily return to their usual stylist!

I would like to go into a clothing store and have someone do the same for me! The most common error? Not knowing how to choose the person you'll trust with your hair. Women who are unhappy with their stylist are also guilty.

There are many categories of stylists, and each has its own type of client. You must find one with whom you can establish a dialogue, communicate well, share your feelings.

The most important thing is the human contact.

I never begin a cut without establishing in detail the length, the color, the shape—it's all about listening and understanding.

▶

"I never begin a cut without establishing in detail the length, the color, the shape . . ."

HOW TO DEVELOP A NEW RANGE

I have thirty years of loyalty to L'Oréal, but I'm more than just a supplier. It has been a partnership, one that guides you and leads you to participate in the evolution of the profession. They are at the top of their research. I worked for two years investigating the expectations of women in order to create a new line of shampoos and hair-care products exclusively for Shu Uemura. This was extremely interesting because we used as a point of departure the work of a makeup artist who wished to reconcile Hollywood glamour with Eastern purity. I will share with you what I have gathered along the way: **When a woman has her stylist in front of her, she is limitless.** Her main expectation: the quality of her hair. And quick results.

I came up with the irrefutable equation: beautiful hair = good care + good products.

Laboratories have managed to invent formulas that simultaneously repair the hair fiber and resolve the problems brought on by the environment. Global warming makes hair drier and drier while, paradoxically, it gets dirty more quickly thanks to pollution. I chose textures that enrich the hair without weighing it down, based on hair type. The ingredients are natural (from camellia to argan) and respectful of the hair's ecosystem. As for perfumes, I want them to be very light—tasteful scents that gradually fade in order to allow room for whatever perfume a woman also wears.

For packaging, I opted for small bottles and tubes in harmony with the sensuality of the texture. I didn't want anything aggressive in the shapes. Most importantly, I wanted them to be easy to use.

FOR SHU UEMURA, I INVENTED HAIR MASSAGE. It's the method of application, which is totally unexpected, that I focused on.

Scalp massages already existed, but this was the first for hair. In a single twenty-minute treatment, you soften hair scale by scale, give it an unexpected suppleness, and return its strength. The goal: a new approach to relaxation. There are ceremonies that last an hour based on techniques inherited from shiatsu. Depending on the needs of the client, we focus on a relaxation massage if the woman is really stressed, or on a detox massage to stimulate and regenerate a tired, damaged scalp.

We have geisha bowls, combs, and paintbrushes, a whole environment based on the art of living in the Japanese style of modernity and calm. A minimalist spirit produces a sublime effect.

Shu Uemura Art of Hair:
An entire line infused with Zen attitude.

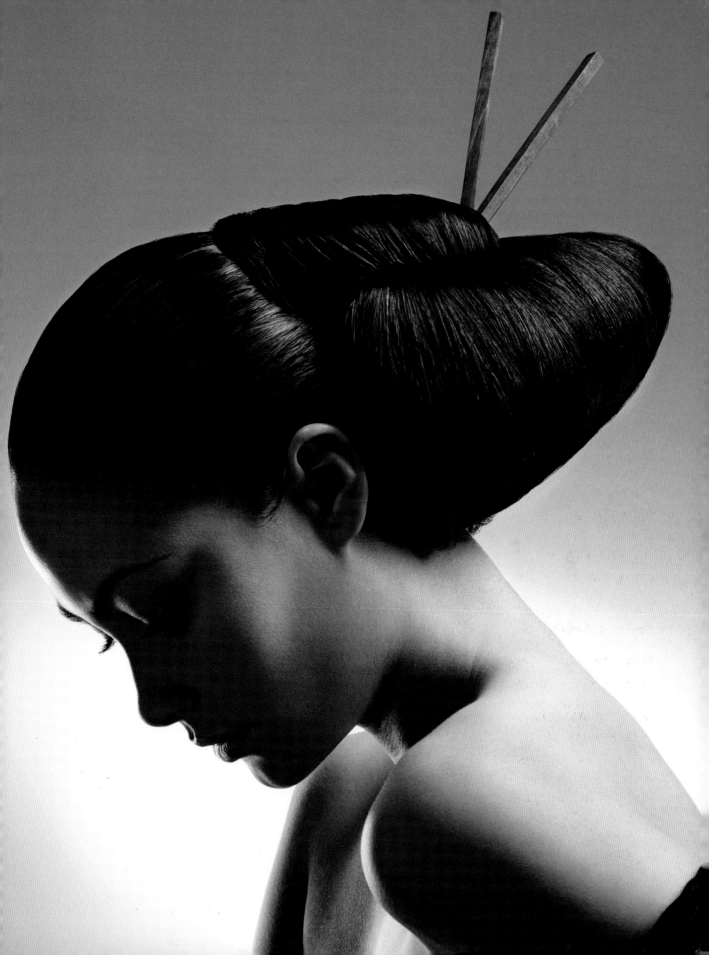

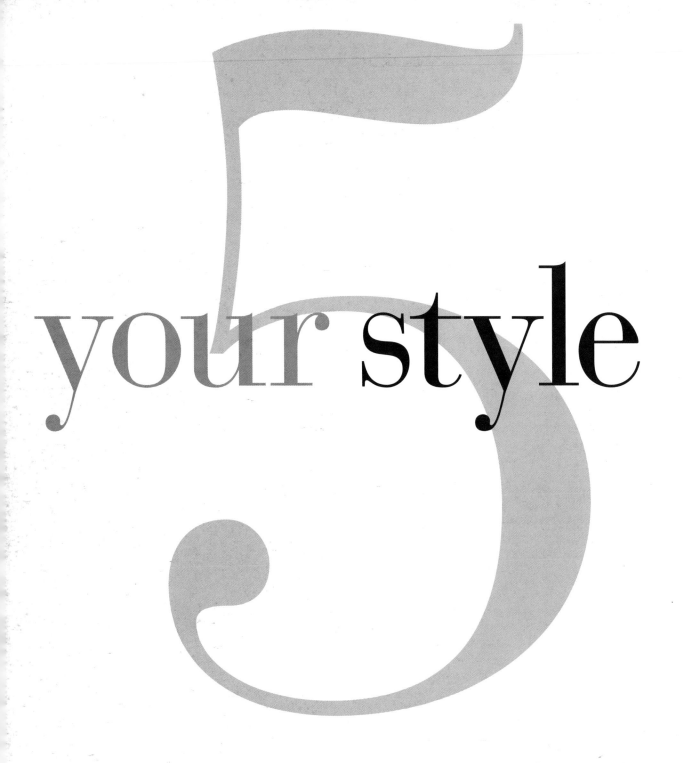

your style

5

SOURCES OF INSPIRATION

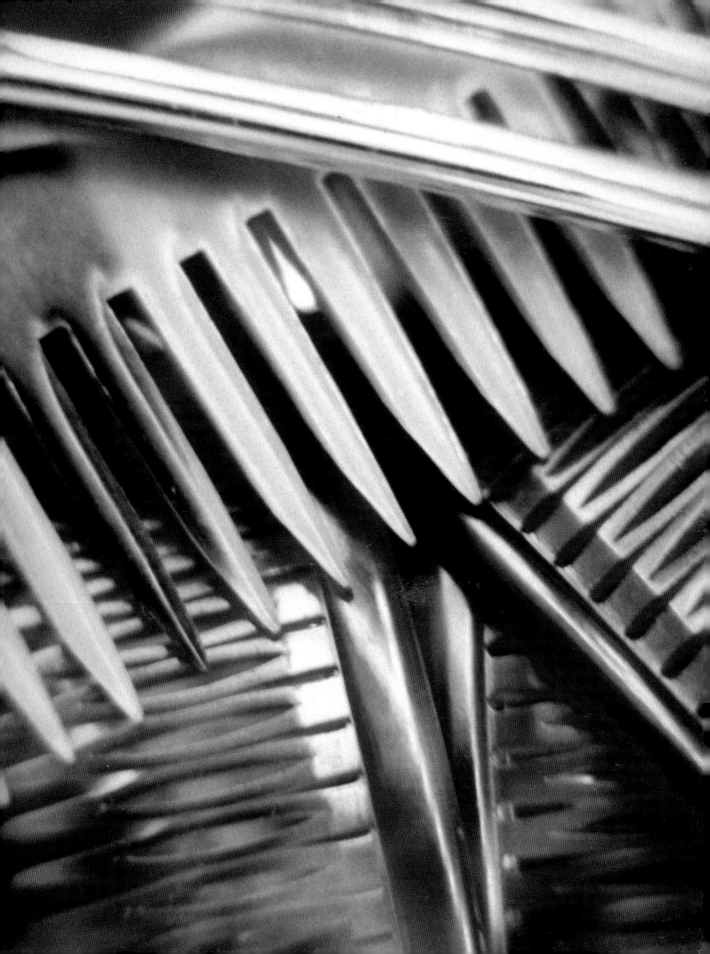

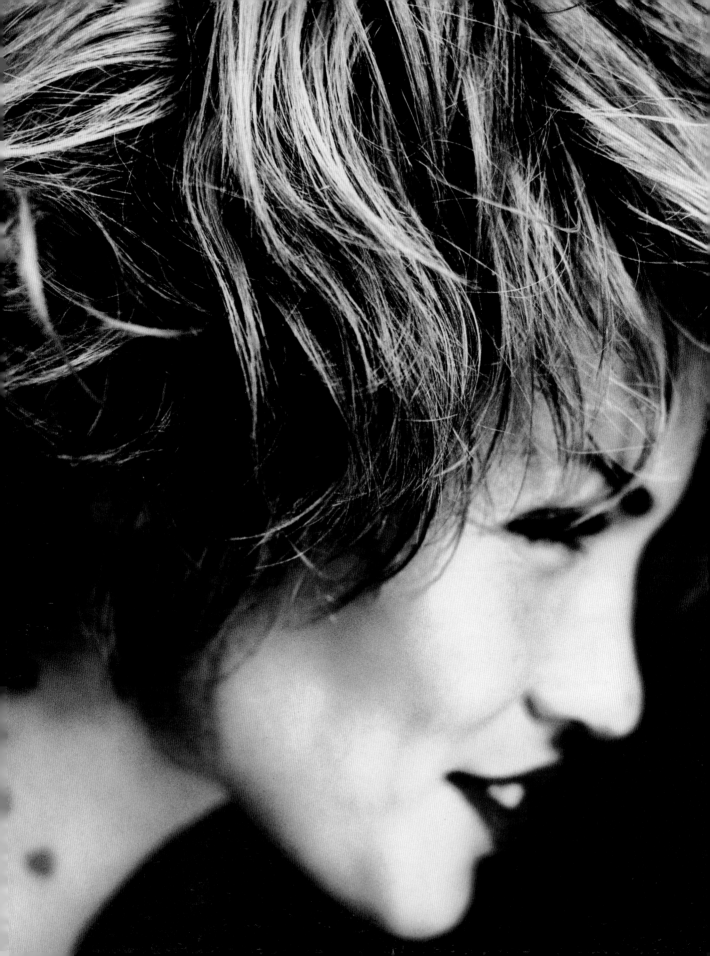

Thinking about your look as a woman of the world...

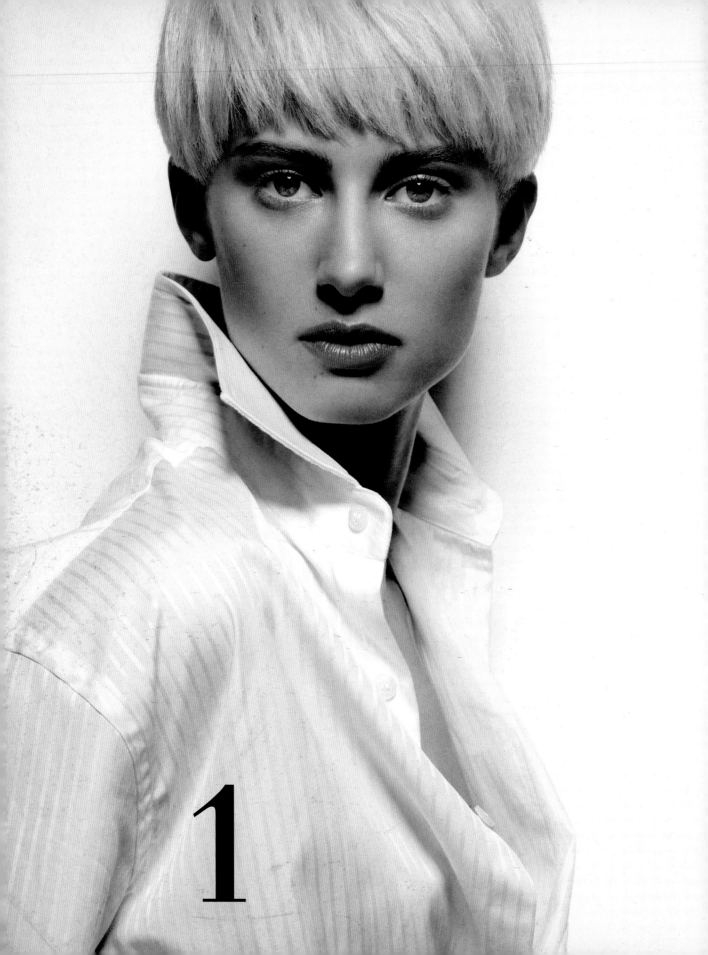

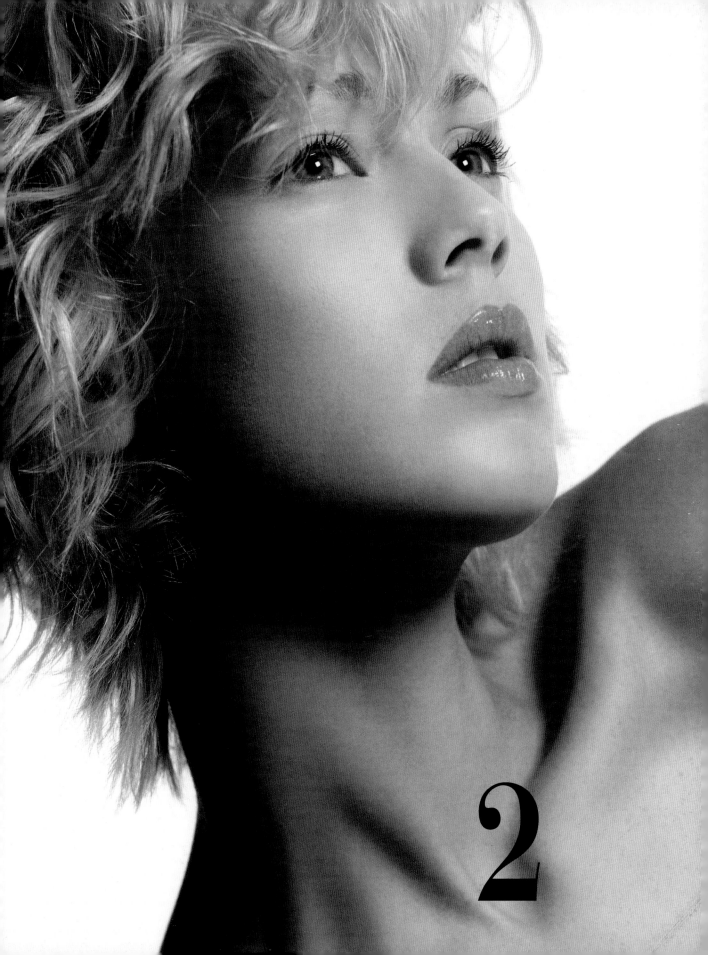

2

Short style: 1 cut 3 looks

A dazzling demonstration in three parts: the undeniable proof that, with a great professional haircut, you can truly do anything!

THREE LOOKS Done by Madeline Cofano.

1 ANDROGYNOUS (page 142) There is a bit of the tomboy in this impeccably smooth and shiny pixie cut with side part. The nape of the neck is bare thanks to a stylist's trick: a mini braid turned up under the hair.

2 FEATHERED (page 143) Little sections of hair blown dry in every direction and then swept forward like little plumes, after having applied a pea-sized amount of heat-styling gel. You can also tuck a section behind your ear and make a three-quarter part.

3 GOLDEN CURLS (at right) Sculpted one by one with a large-barrel curling iron for softer curls after working some styling mousse through the hair.

ADVICE FROM A STYLIST
Curls should be worked like knitting: One curl forward, one curl back, alternating direction one after the other. A natural effect is guaranteed!

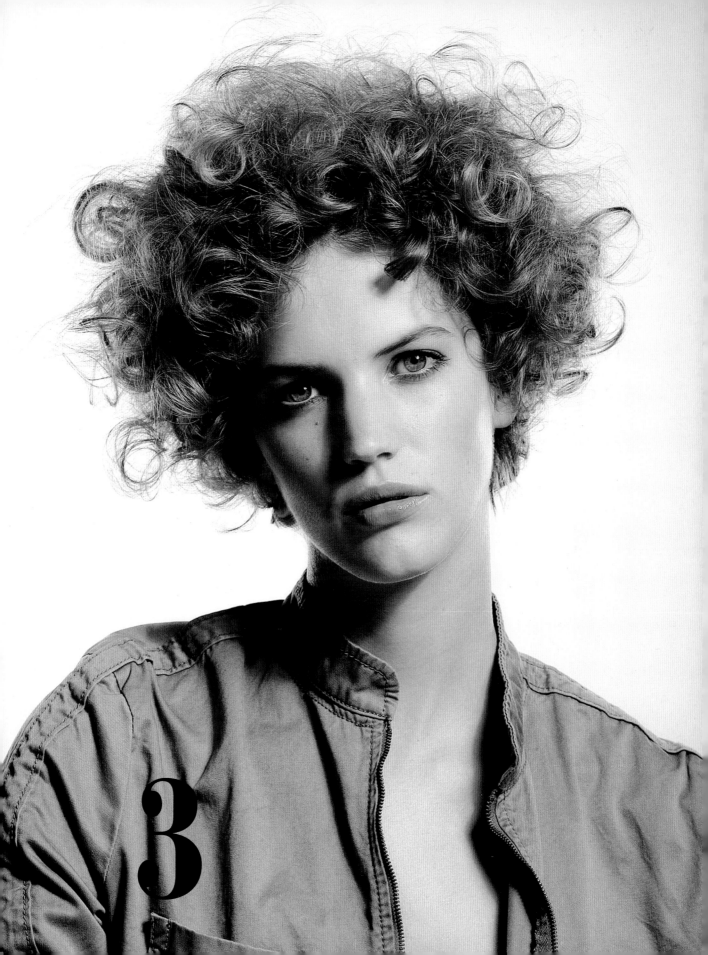

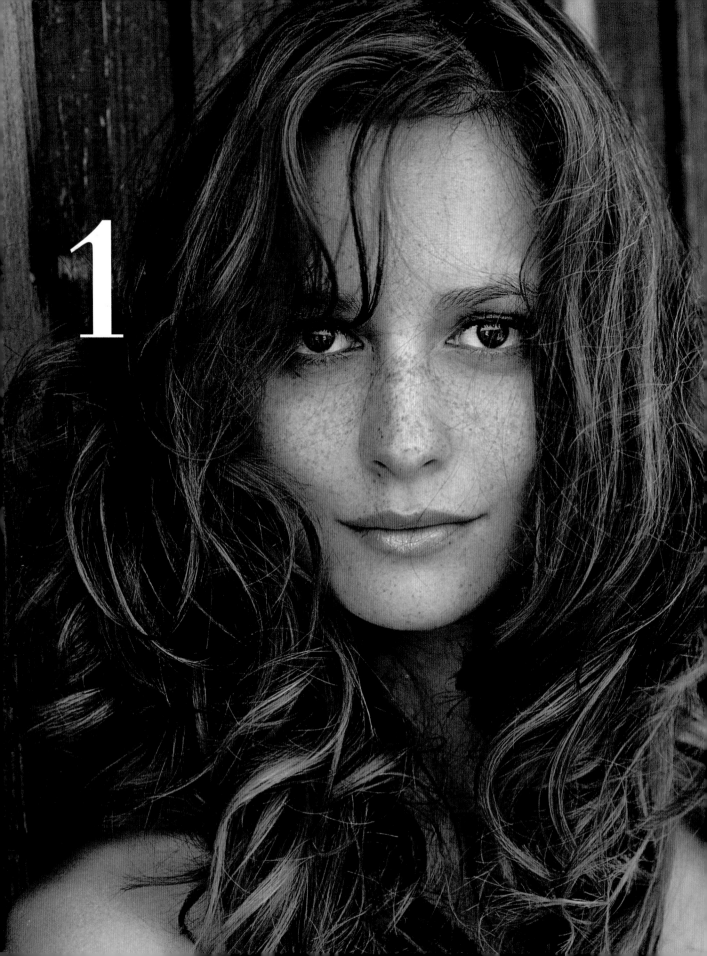

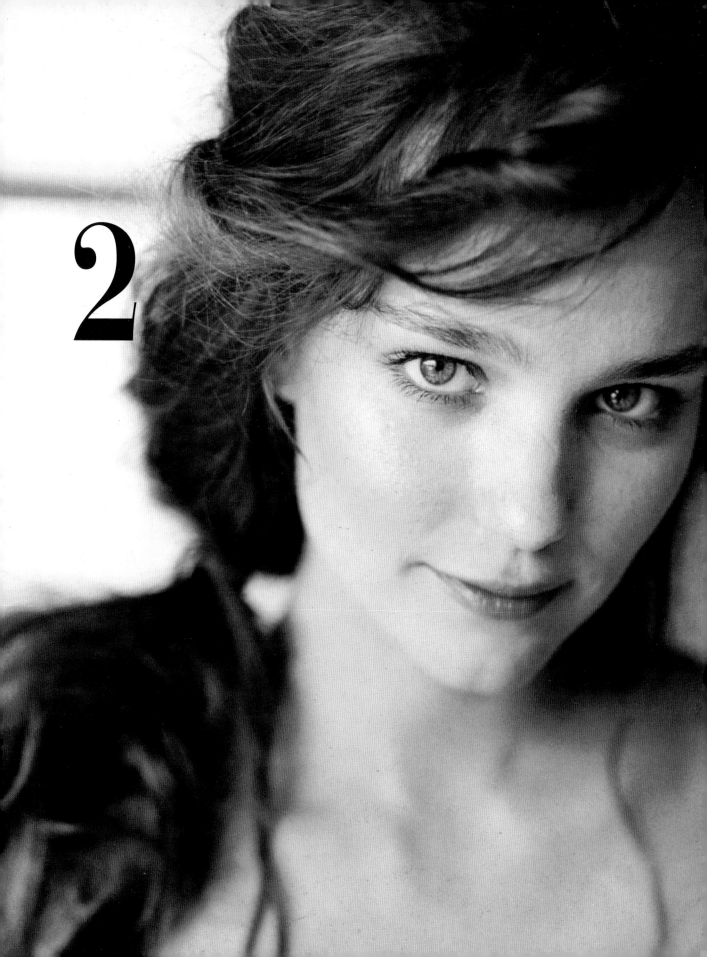

2

Long style: 1 cut 3 looks

Shoulder length and long hair, or even extensions, allow for many different looks. Here are three very popular ones to get you started.

SHOCKING TRIO A very adaptable style centered on long bangs and long layers, designed by Max Laffite.

1 GIRLY CURLS (page 146) The softness of well-defined waves gives this style plenty of femininity. Prepare your hair with a mousse designed for curls and dry with a diffuser while you scrunch with your hand.

2 TIE ME UP (page 147) A chic, urban version of a ponytail, worn low and off-center. An elastic band is hidden under a lock of hair wrapped around it and held with a bobby pin, leaving a section free on the side.

3 SUPERSTAR EXTENSIONS (at right) A very '60s style, with bangs slightly curled under, ends layered and everything incredibly shiny. The effect is obtained using a styling lotion, drying with a paddle brush, then finishing the ends with a smoothing iron.

ADVICE FROM A STYLIST
The ponytail shown with this style can easily be transformed into a chignon. All you need to do is twist the ends and fasten them with a few bobby pins.

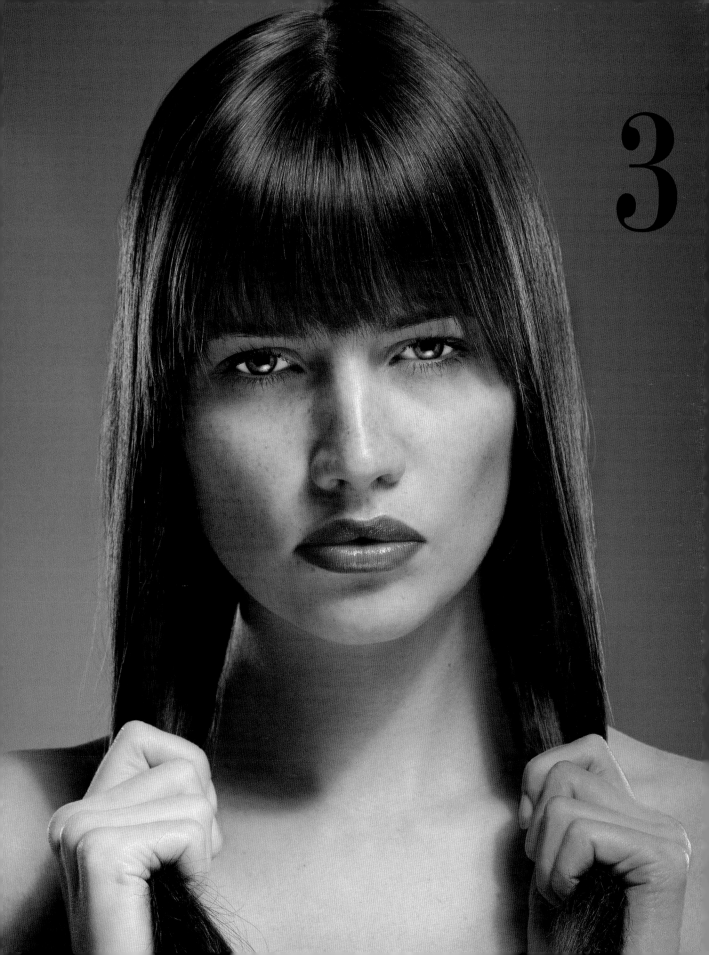

3

It's all about seduction!

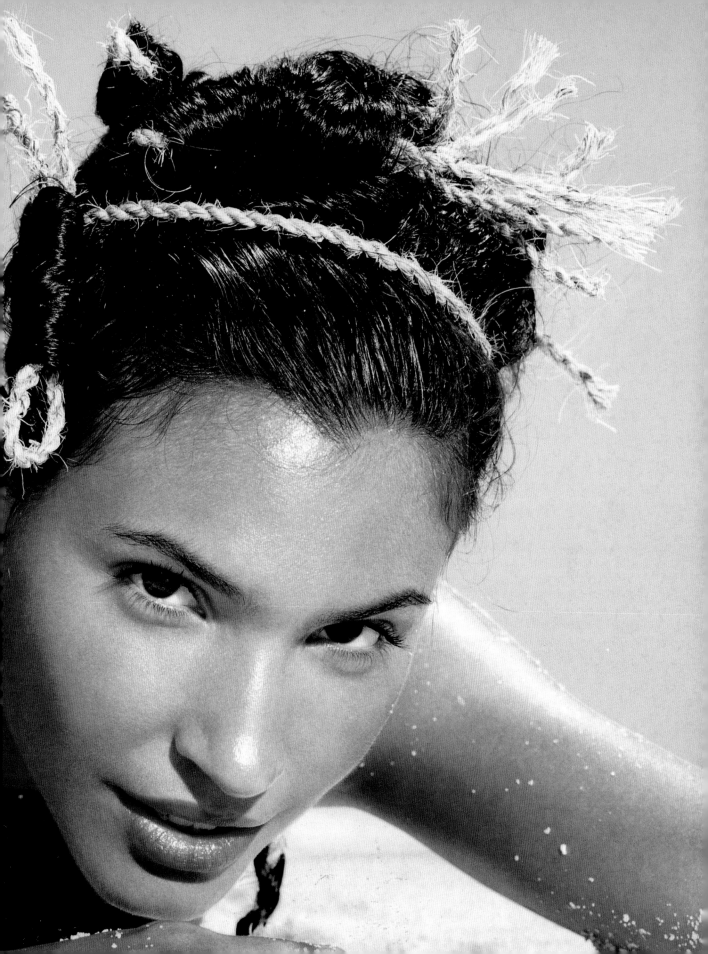

Beautiful bangs!

They can do anything—frame the face, add mystery, but also hide an irregular hairline or wrinkles on your forehead. They can even be pushed back for a change of scenery!

ADVICE FROM STYLIST MADEILINE COFANO

YES TO BANGS . . .

- If you have a small forehead (cut bangs straight across at eyebrow level for a guaranteed optical illusion)
- If you have a broad or large chin
- If you have a strong profile
- If you have high cheekbones

YES, BUT . . .

- For oval faces, rounded bangs work best
- For square faces, bangs parted to the side work best

NO TO BANGS . . .

- If you have a larger forehead, a side part is better
- If your hairline starts far back on your forehead, a tapered part looks better
- If your face is very square, bangs tend to make it more serene

1 THE '60S (facing page, left top and bottom) This is quintessential retro look: long, straight, and thick, beginning very high on the crown and following a perfect path down the forehead, ending just above the ears. **To push them back:** try the spiky Mohawk. Part the hair from your bangs into a triangle, tease it a bit at the roots, and begin to form your Mohawk with spiky ends. Twirl locks of hair into rosettes, using bobby pins or flat barrettes to secure them to the scalp. Allow the ends to remain free, forming the spikes.

2 WILD AND WAVY (facing page, right top and bottom) These extremely long bangs are given a lift by using the blowdryer to avoid a weighed-down, heavy look. Scrunch volumizing mousse into your hair and then finish with a shine spray. **To tie them back:** Show off your face by pulling your hair all the way back, as done here with a hairband by Odile Gilbert, with or without a ponytail.

UPKEEP Having bangs requires maintenance, which can be demanding. **For straight hair,** you must use a blowdryer every morning. **For curly hair,** spray bangs with a bit of mineral water, shape with your fingers, and allow them to air-dry without brushing (otherwise, they will frizz).

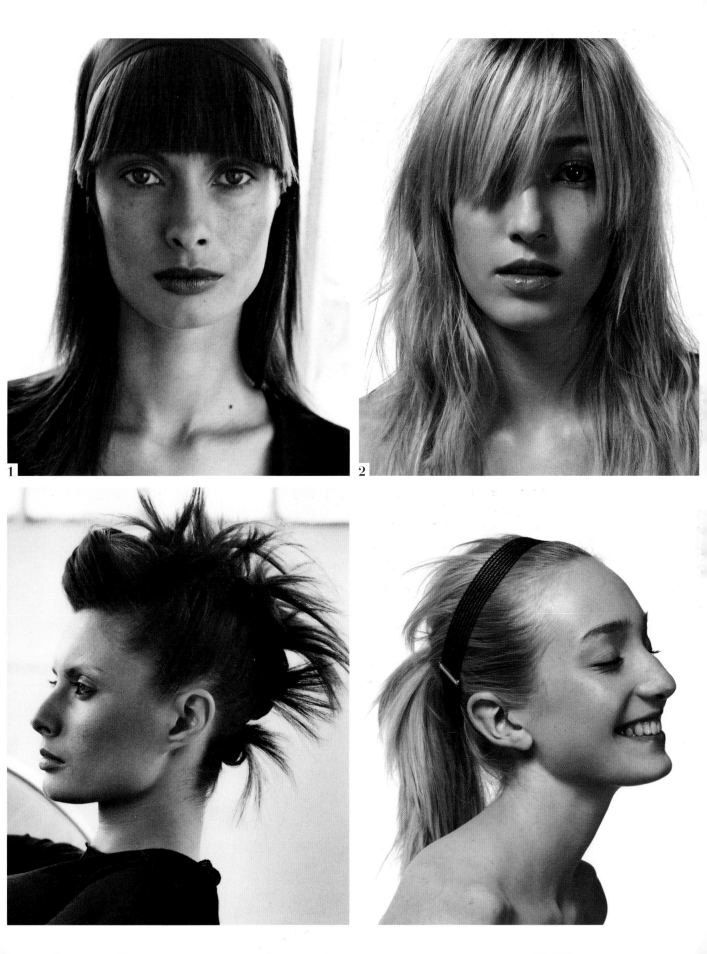

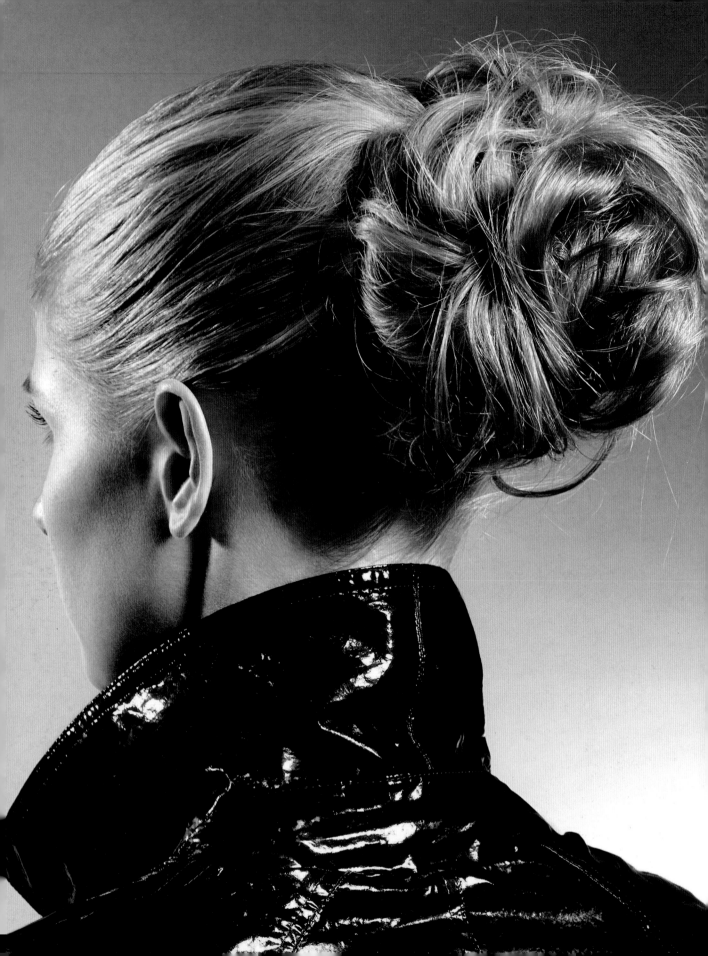

Chignon how-to

A chignon can lend evening elegance to a little black dress or allow you to bare your shoulders to the first rays of the summer sun. Instantly chic, it lets you change your look by accessorizing it however you wish. Perfectly pretty!

1 **STRAIGHTEN WITH A FLATIRON** beginning at the nape and finishing with the hair in the front. Take one-inch sections and slowly smooth them with the iron from root to ends.

2 **GATHER HAIR** into a ponytail positioned where you want to place your chignon. We place ours at the top of the crown.

3 **ROLL** hair into four or five large hot rollers to add volume.

4 **TWIST** your hair tightly to make the base of the chignon, then twirl the remaining hair around a bit more loosely. Fasten ends with bobby pins.

5 **LOOSEN** a few strands with the tail of a comb or with a pencil (around your hairline, on the sides, at your nape) to avoid looking too severe. A mist of shine spray and you'll be ready to go!

HELPFUL HINT Hair that has just been washed is not as easy to pull back into a chignon: to get a better result, use some mousse to give hair better hold.

ADVICE FROM STYLIST BERNARD FRIBOULET
Hair not long enough? Temporary extensions made of natural hair can be attached in twenty minutes and can stay in for three days. Use soft, gentle, elastic bands to avoid breaking hairs.

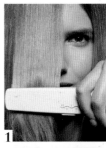
1

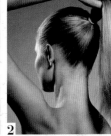
2

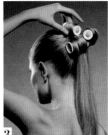
3

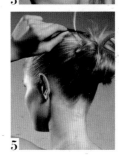
4

5

Cool, regal braids!

Irresistible in all their forms, from the most simple to the most elaborate, braids allow you to look neat and tidy once you learn the technique.

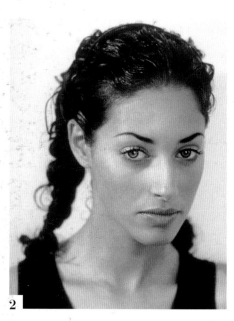

2

ADVICE FROM STYLIST BRUNO SILVANI
Use transparent elastic bands that blend into your hair color, and "grease" them (with sunscreen, for example) so they don't damage hair and will be easy to remove later.

NATURALLY FEMININE

1 IN BACK—the classic revisited. It can hang to your nape or down to the small of your back, depending on the length of your hair. You can also boost the effect with the help of hair extensions. For this look, gather your hair loosely at the crown and make a part, starting at the top of your head. Rather than dividing into three sections right away, start by working two sections, passing one over the other. Then divide hair into three sections and braid tightly, finishing with an elastic band, leaving an inch or two free at the end. Add a flower or ribbon— your decorative options are endless!

2 PIGTAIL BRAIDS Use the same technique described above, but separate the hair with a center part and begin the braids a bit higher, above the ear.

3 TWISTED CORN ROWS Beginning at your hairline and working toward the back, make many little braids (it's easier if you have someone help you). When you are done, wind the ends around your head and secure with hairpins.

4 HELEN OF TROY First, push hair back and secure with a tight headband. Next, take a few pieces and braid them in the cornrow style before attaching them in a figure-eight shape using bobby pins (bend them slightly to resemble a fish hook). Interlace the braids and leave some pieces of hair free.

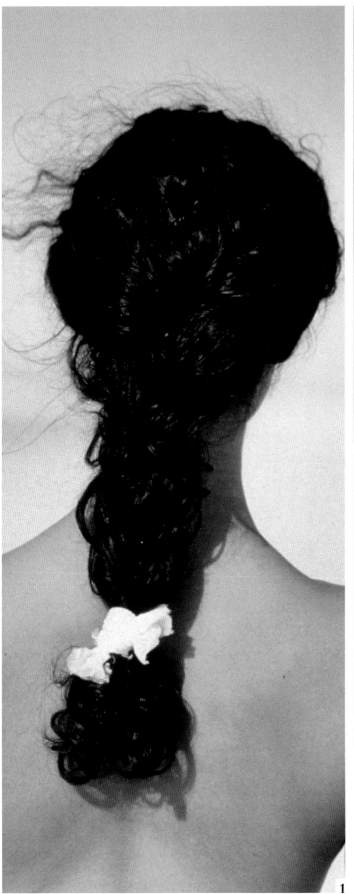

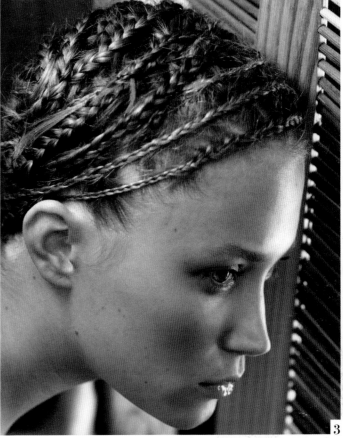

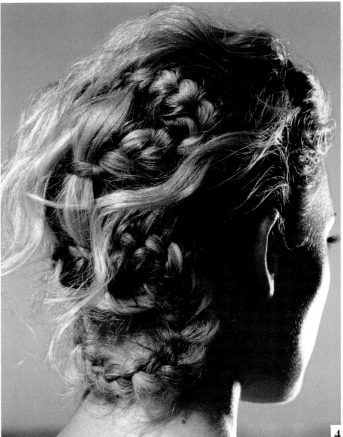

Celeb-style makeovers

How do you bring out your best with just a few snips of the scissors and strokes of the brush? Here are six before-and-after stories featuring star-worthy makeovers by pro stylists.

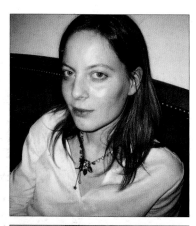

MICKAELA MAKEOVER BY JEAN-MARC MANIATIS (left)

The Cut

We balanced out her oval face with a few highlighted wisps that softened the look of a large forehead. We kept the length, just added layers for volume.

The Color

We abandoned the chestnut brown for brighter blonde highlights, obtained in two steps using three different shades.

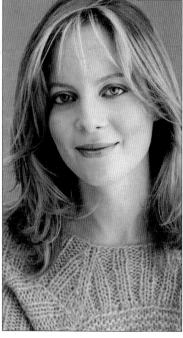

CÉLINE MAKEOVER BY BERNARD FRIBOULET (far right)

The Cut

The unanimous decision: A short cut to replace her plain style and fine, lifeless hair. The miraculous result: Her natural curls find a new life and expose the pretty line of her neck.

The Color

From mousy brown she becomes a luminous blonde with sunkissed highlights.

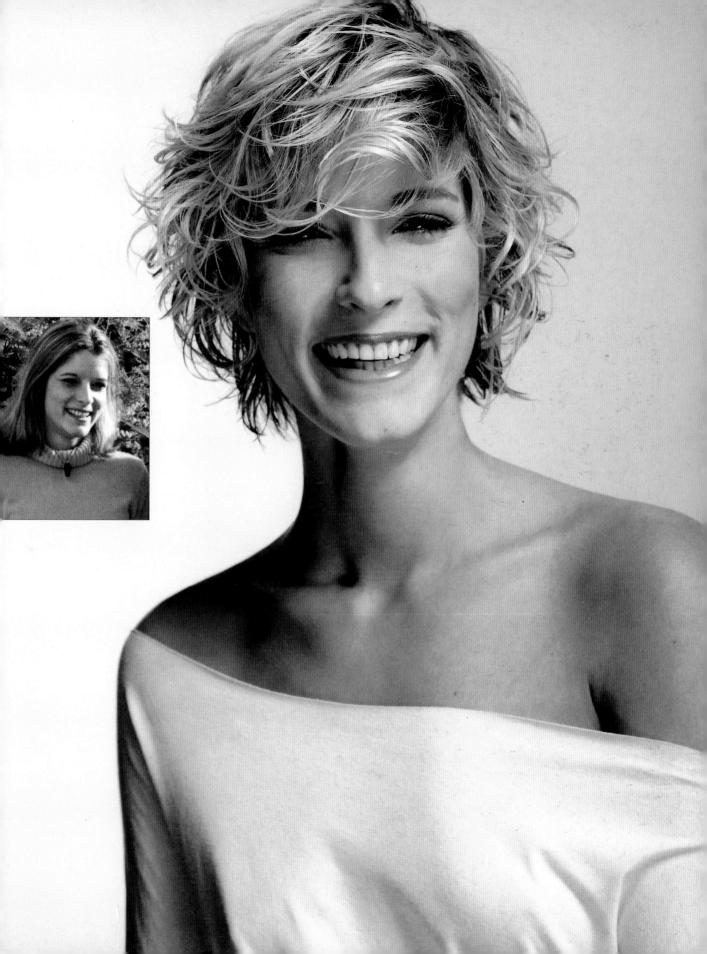

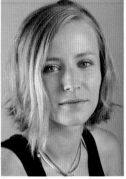

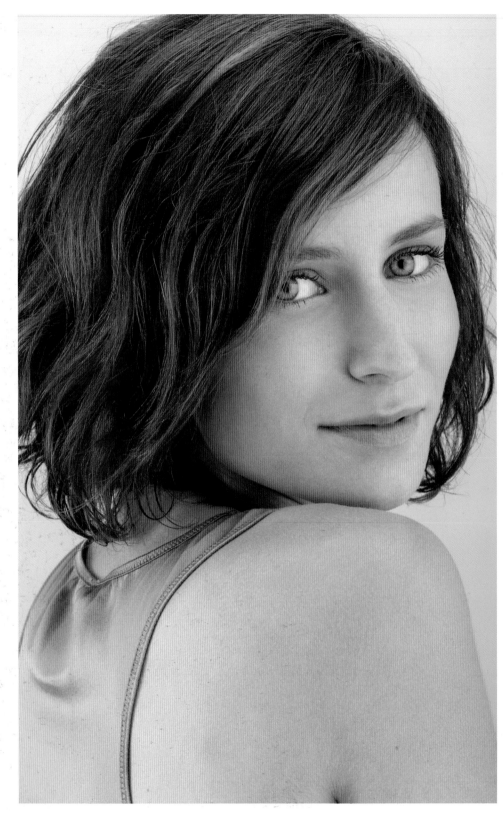

CHRISTELLE MAKEOVER BY ALEXANDRE ZOUARI

The Cut

A sculpted shape that starts at the nape and gets progressively longer to combine volume and softness.

The Color

A mix of light golden red (close to Venetian blonde) and a very warm, richly pigmented copper, with large sections "woven in" in an irregular way to emphasize the cut and highlight the movement of her hair.

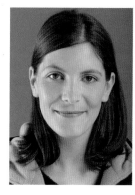

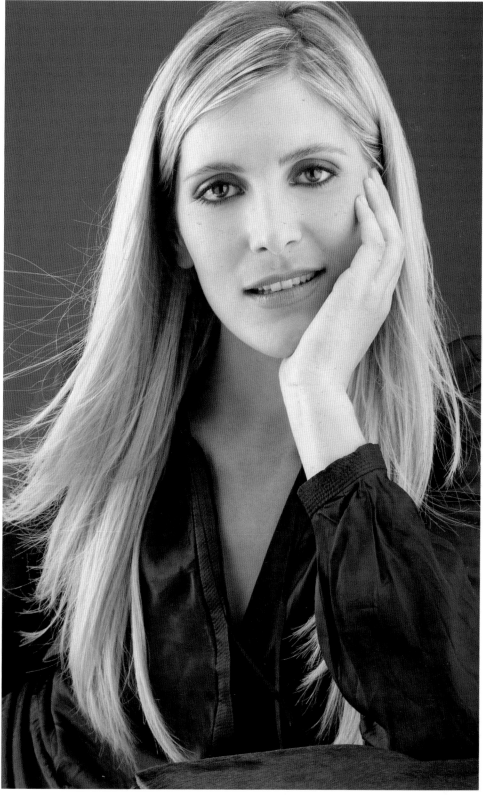

MARYLINE MAKEOVER BY MADEILINE COFANO AND CHRISTOPHE ROBIN

The Cut

Hair extensions offer a bit of a rock-and-roll effect, helped along by drying with a large round brush.

The Color

This was a very specialized task, which preserved the darker shades at the roots, and added small sections of golden blonde and larger sections of almost-platinum blonde.

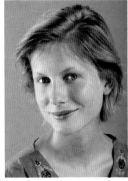

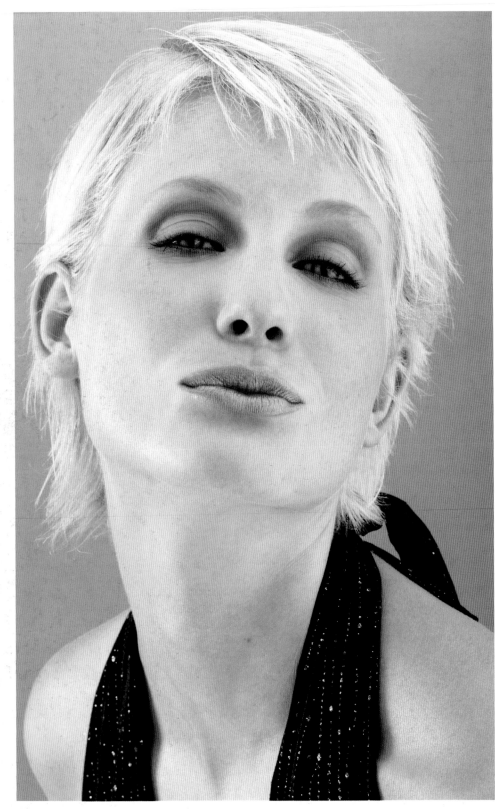

ASIA MAKEOVER BY JEAN-MARC MANIATIS

The Cut

This shag cut is done with scissors, leaving "longer, wispy sections at the nape to soften, feminize, and do away with her tomboy look." Hair is swept to the side without making a part, with little uneven sections overlapping and forming a soft crown.

The Color

Very light, slightly golden blonde, finished with sections of platinum on top to highlight the cut and give it depth.

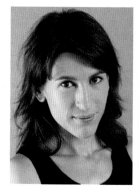

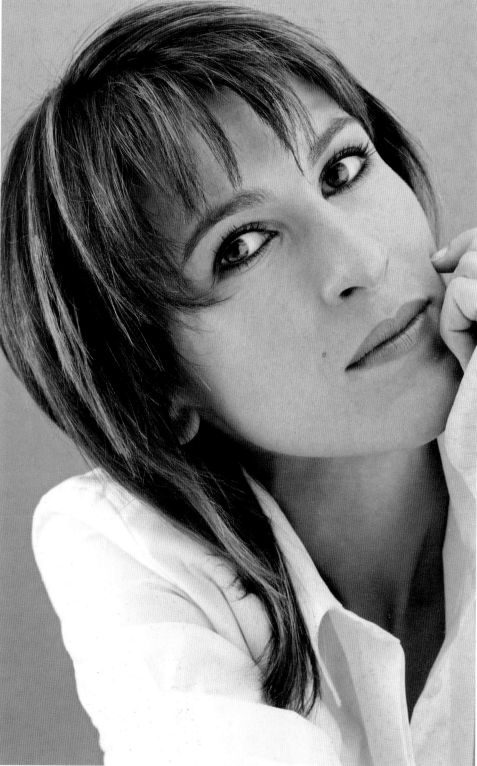

LAURENCE MAKEOVER BY ALEXANDRE ZOUARI

The Cut

Hair is layered in the direction of growth so that, when styled, it will look natural. We did not change the length, but the layers added volume and gave it lightness.

The Color

A tone-on-tone color base to cover the gray and concentrate pigment on the ends to highlight the movement of the cut.

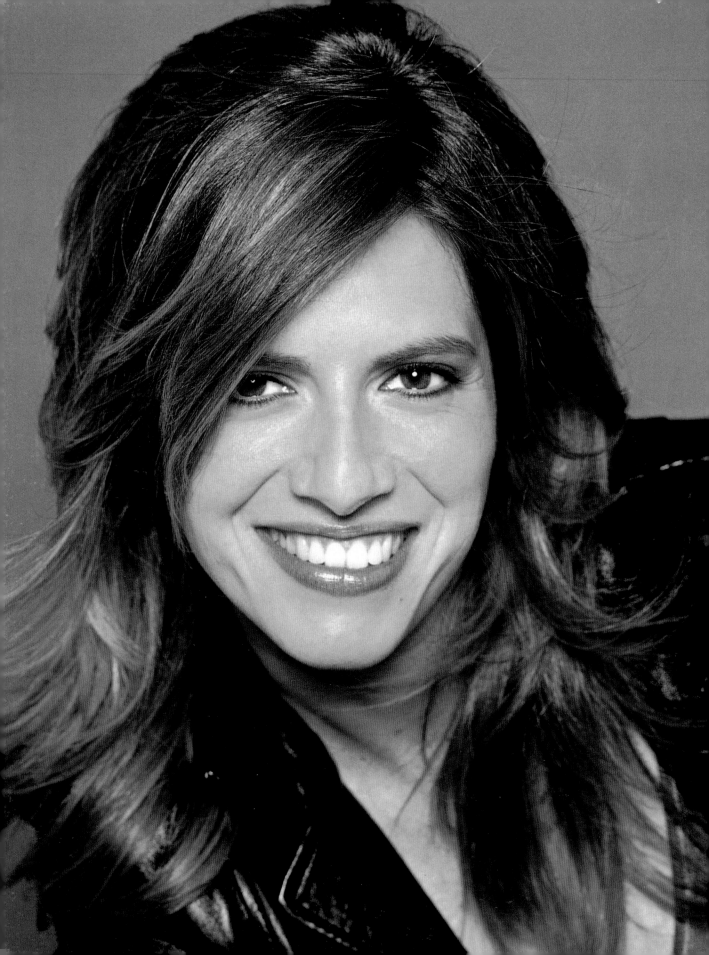

Change your appearance: The remedy

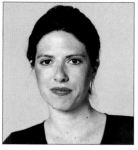

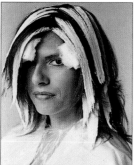

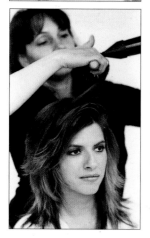

THE STYLE TO DE-EMPHASIZE DELPHINE'S NOSE BY MADELEINE COFANO

Before

Delphine's nose is part of her personality, so we don't want to cover it up, but simply re-balance the overall appearance of her face. Her hair was too long, too heavy, almost always pulled back, which choked her face. And despite a beautiful base of amber brown, her color was a bit too uniform.

The Cut

Long layers were cut section by section to taper the ends and give them a feathery lightness. So as not to dwarf her forehead, a highlighted, side-parted bang brings her profile into view.

The Color

Color used in twos or threes emphasizes the cut and blends the ends by playing with shadow and light. The hairline is brushed with golden honey, weaving in tones of malt that will "disappear" into the rest of the hair. The result is a sumptuous sunkissed look.

THE BEST APPROACH

Fully analyze and accept yourself without ever erasing your personality: Highlighting your perceived "flaws" can sometimes be the best way to camouflage them!

TIPS FROM A STYLIST
HIDING AN IMPERFECTION

- For a large, thin nose: keep forehead clear
- To soften your profile: side-swept bangs to create volume and softness
- For a strong jaw: wispy bangs
- For a thick neck: soft, tapered ends

ADVICE FROM COLORIST LAETITIA GUENAOU
OPTICAL ILLUSIONS CREATED WITH COLOR

- For a round face: A few darker pieces create shadows that will highlight and soften
- To lengthen your silhouette: Lighten the very top of your crown
- To look younger: Choose golden and honey shades

Tricks for looking younger

A stylist's tools may just be the source of the fountain of youth!
Color can stop time, while scissors gently snip away the years!

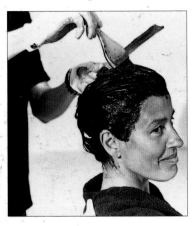

MARIE-MARTINE MAKEOVER BY ALEXANDRE ZOUARI

Before

She wears a long braid in back, which, although impeccable, is a bit severe, especially with her dark chestnut hair that has no highlights.

The Cut

We gave her the famous feathered cut to achieve lightness at the crown. It's the perfect way to show off another facet of your personality.

The Color

Successful color is the best anti-ager! Here we show lightening (left) applied with a brush so there are no roots, providing incredible luminosity.

THE BEST APPROACH

Balance between the two extremes: Don't try to play the teenage girl, but don't fall into the role of the schoolmarm, either (i.e., with a severe chignon). Anything goes, thanks to the art of the stylist, but everything depends on the nature of your hair.

ADVICE FROM STYLIST ALEXANDRE ZOUARI
HOW TO LOOK TEN YEARS YOUNGER

- Straight hair: a layered bob to show off and brighten the face
- Fine hair: short wispy layers to give the impression of volume
- Curly hair: a gently layered bob, but avoid going too short!

ADVICE FROM COLORIST JOHN NOLLET
FOUNTAIN OF YOUTH
Soft highlights in gentle tones not too far from your natural color will hide gray hair and create a bit of contrast. This will give depth to blondes and redheads.

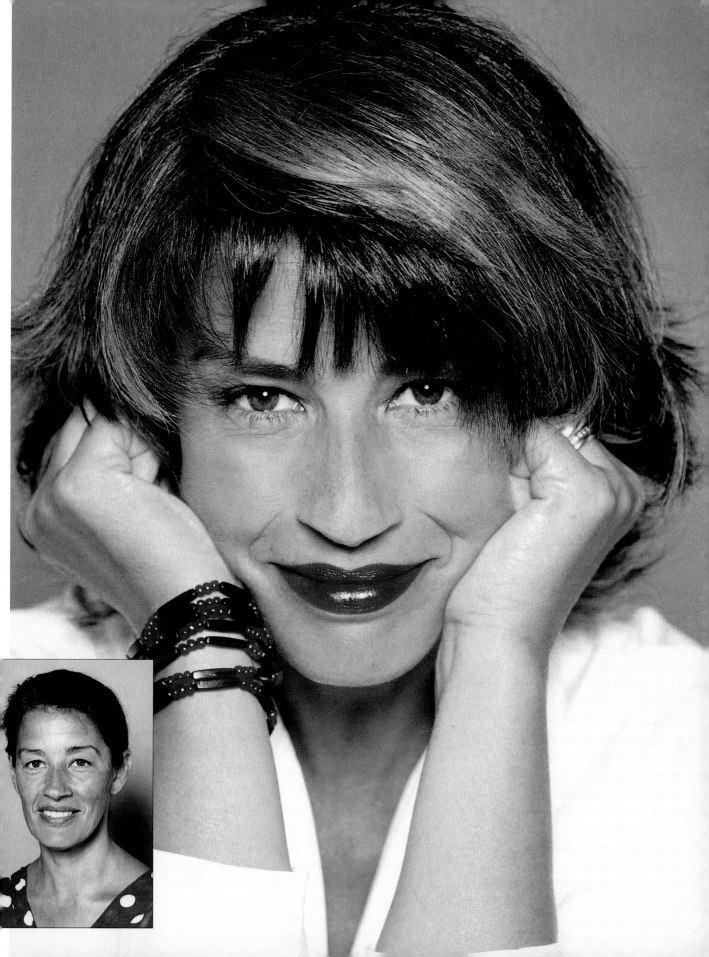

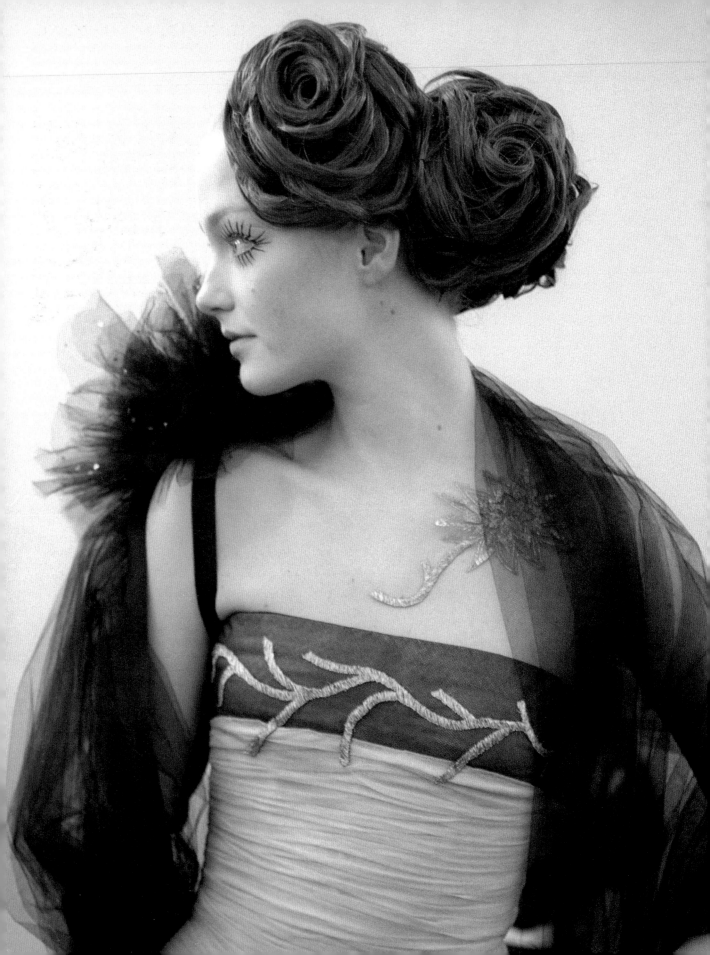

Odile Gilbert

Stylist

Over the years, this virtuoso has created the most remarkable hair designs for haute couture as well as ready-to-wear fashion shows. In her hands, hair is transformed into a work of art—like in Sofia Coppola's film Marie Antoinette.

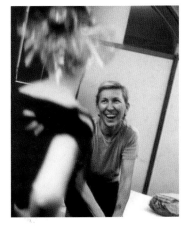

"My motto? Anything is possible! Whatever your hair type! That's the true magic of styling!"

To be the first stylist to have been awarded the title Knight of Arts and Letters is a true recognition in the profession. The other is my book, *Her Style, Hair by Odile Gilbert,* the only book to bring together great photographers, 35 of the best in 350 pages. What has meant so much in my life so far has been meetings with photographers Richard Avedon and Helmut Newton, Irving Penn and Herb Ritts, Peter Lindbergh, Jean-Baptiste Mondino, Paolo Roversi. Designers such as Karl Lagerfeld, Christian Lacroix, John Galliano, and Jean-Paul Gaultier.

THE IMAGES ARE NECESSARILY POWERFUL: WITH EACH ONE YOU ENTER A DIFFERENT UNIVERSE—THAT OF A CREATOR, WITH INCREDIBLE EXCHANGES OF ENERGY.

Sofia Coppola called me after seeing my book, asking me to be the stylist for her film's queen. This was obviously a different way of working, assuming the role of a historian or documentary maker. There was important research to do on the fashion of the era, but it was also important to highlight her modernity—**Kirsten Dunst was the only person in the entire cast who never wore a wig.** I spent many days on the set, with a close team member taking my place when I could not be there. ▶

"To adapt to each client, to make them happy before making yourself happy, that is essential."

It's a tough career, but it must be my Brittany strength—I left home for Paris at 17—that helped me to accept myself in this universe. And almost immediately I met with a master: Bruno Pittini. He was one of those exceptional people who gives you, along with the love of the profession, what no school could teach—a way of opening your eyes and learning how to see. I spent ten years at his side before creating Atelier 68 in Paris.

You become a stylist the day you realize that you are capable of anything, of styling the entire world, from a child to an elderly person, giving them a style that is an exceptional success for that individual. **It's a universal language.**

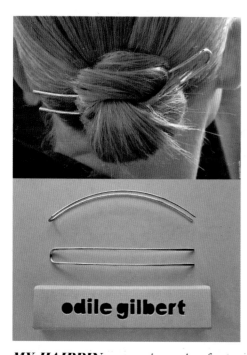

MY HAIRPIN, a true invention for women: It conforms to the shape of the head and comes in three sizes so that everyone will be able to make a chignon. Catherine Deneuve only needs one to do hers!

I have been all over the world, thanks to my profession. There are no borders in this career—there are photo shoots and fashion shows in Paris, New York, Tokyo, Los Angeles, and Milan. Within twenty years I had been everywhere. I am a pioneer. I have had the opportunity to practice my trade how I please—it's a choice, an opening of the spirit. In France, we have haute couture, a unique heritage, but today, fashion is international: We work with all races, all cultures—it's brilliant.

AT A FASHION SHOW, I AM THE HEAD OF THE BACKSTAGE HAIR, so I determine, along with the designer, a look that will then be created by a team of nearly thirty stylists behind the scenes. I could never style fifty models all at the same time! What has changed is the way of life for women. You have to be everywhere at the same time.

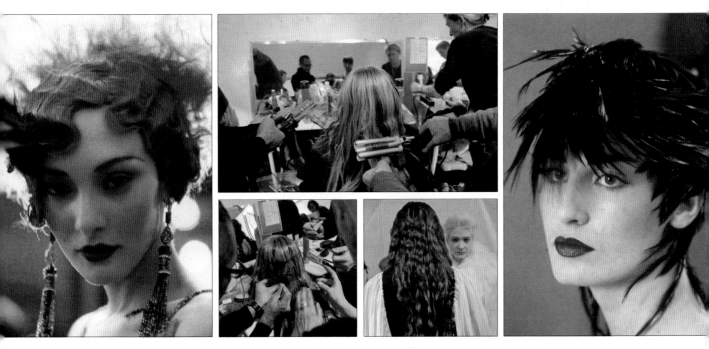

A STAR IS BACK(STAGE)! At the top of the platform, among these sublime birds of paradise, Gilbert manages a dizzying ballet in which dozens of stars make their entrance on the runway (at center, Ann Demeulemeester's fashion show).

THE REPERCUSSION: YOU ALWAYS NEED TO BE STYLED. Of course, there are things you can do yourself everyday. Taking care of yourself has become very important. There is beauty at every age. And I don't say this just to make women happy! Today Sharon Stone could have a beauty contract, or Jane Fonda, who is over 60 years old! Experience counts, and that's something new. We're more flexible nowadays, anything goes. We have the right to have long hair at 70 if that makes us happy—and why not make the most of hair extensions.

EVERY DAY, YOU CAN DO SOMETHING TO CARE FOR YOUR HAIR. But when it comes to a cut or color, you always need to go to a salon.

Makeup is very important, but hair truly cannot be overlooked.

STYLISTS ARE ARTISANS BECAUSE WE WORK WITH OUR HANDS.

It is a very technical profession. There is chemistry, and it takes a long time to learn—you don't become a stylist overnight. It requires years of experience. Then you must assimilate it and forget it (visual and artistic work requires it) to then be able to directly enter into a symbiosis with the cut, the style, the human approach. Every day you touch someone you do not know, and that is the strangest ▶

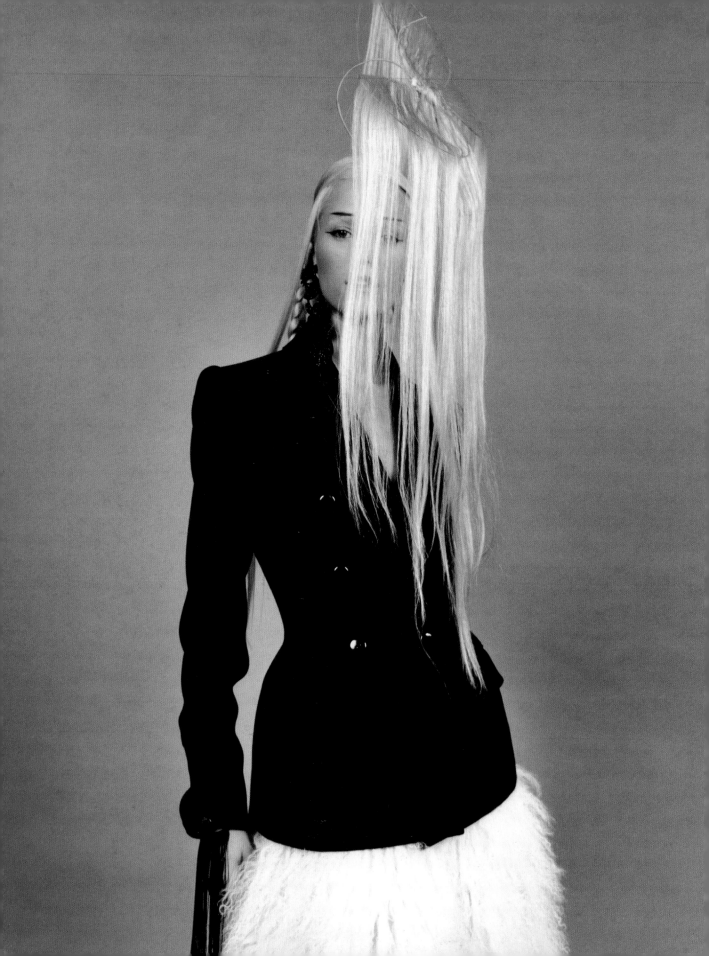

"You have the right to have long hair at 70, thanks to extensions!"

thing. And as a stylist, you need to help them bring out the best in themselves. Each person has his or her own beauty, and it's up to us to allow it to emerge.

A mistake can sometimes be interesting—but I can't prevent myself from fixing it. When I look at a woman, it's with a professional eye. Most often, it's simply a matter of proportion. That's where a stylist can intervene. We can find what you can do better, based on face shape or hair quality—but it's truly case by case. Everyone is different, and there is not one ideal hairstyle. The secret is to find the perfect balance. You must respect the nature of hair, its texture, but also know how to look at someone without being influenced by trends. You must always adapt to the hair, the face, the person—and always make them happy before making yourself happy, that is essential. In total, it's about drawing out and emphasizing what nature would have given us.

GOOD HAIR CARE GIVES YOU SHINE, THE MIRROR EFFECT—it's easy if you're a professional! Good hair care has become fundamental, it has evolved so much. The majority of women have highlights or colored hair, and these demand daily maintenance.

We work all the time, we're stressed out, and hair care has become a little, indispensable retreat. We are looking for organic and natural in an era where a product cleans at the same time as it embellishes.

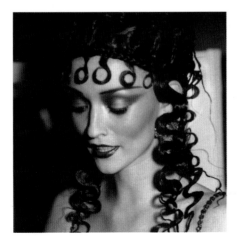

Hair nutrition, specific vitamins, and treatments work, but take a long time, a year at least, to show results. You can't wait even fifteen days for results if your hair is very fine! But the miracle product that will make your hair really thick is not yet on the market—its inventor would be a millionaire!

HOW TO FIND YOUR COLOR A good color is one that matches your complexion: It awakens your skin and gives it brightness. Not every shade will work for everyone.

▶

"The first adornment for a woman, before jewelry, is her hair."

Finding the right BLONDE is very important. Even among those who were born blonde, like me, whose blonde is naturally dark, lighten it. This requires permanent upkeep, because you will be intervening chemically, but the products have also evolved considerably with healthy dyes. You really need a stylist for this, for maintenance and highlights.

For BRUNETTES, move toward warm colors. All the shades of brown, from light to dark, work very well. Black hair is rare, but they also love to warm it up.

Becoming a REDHEAD is enormously popular. I love red hair on very pale skin. It's so pretty on supermodels Karen Elson or Lily Cole, but also on actresses like Julianne Moore.

Whatever the color, whether it's blonde, brown, or red, I love to make it a bit golden. I love highlights. The sun can help you achieve natural highlights—just be sure to use products to protect it from too much exposure.

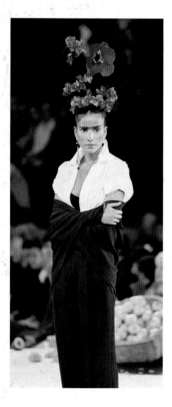

It's always best to go lighter as you get older. I adore gray hair, a woman with completely gray hair, I find that magical. It's always best to accept your gray. With age, beyond color, you have to be gentle. I am always fascinated by older women who still have that quality of seduction to them, that dignity. It's impressive when women continue making that effort.

Hair extensions allow for incredible manes, even if you have fine or short hair. But it is a delicate and time-consuming task.

DON'T KEEP THE SAME STYLE ALL YOUR LIFE! But if you do, and it still works, you can be happy. You have the right to try different things, it's fun to find your look.

Haircuts should be adapted to your lifestyle. The work of the stylist, like that of a tailor, is to find a style that will fall into place nicely on its own.

We all desire thick, luxurious hair.

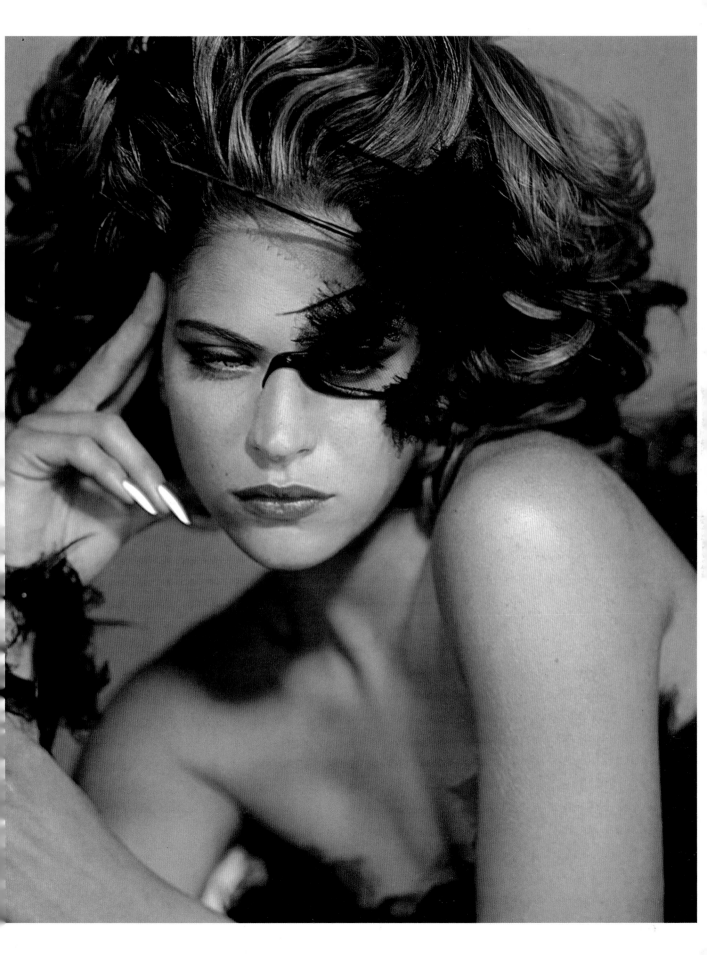

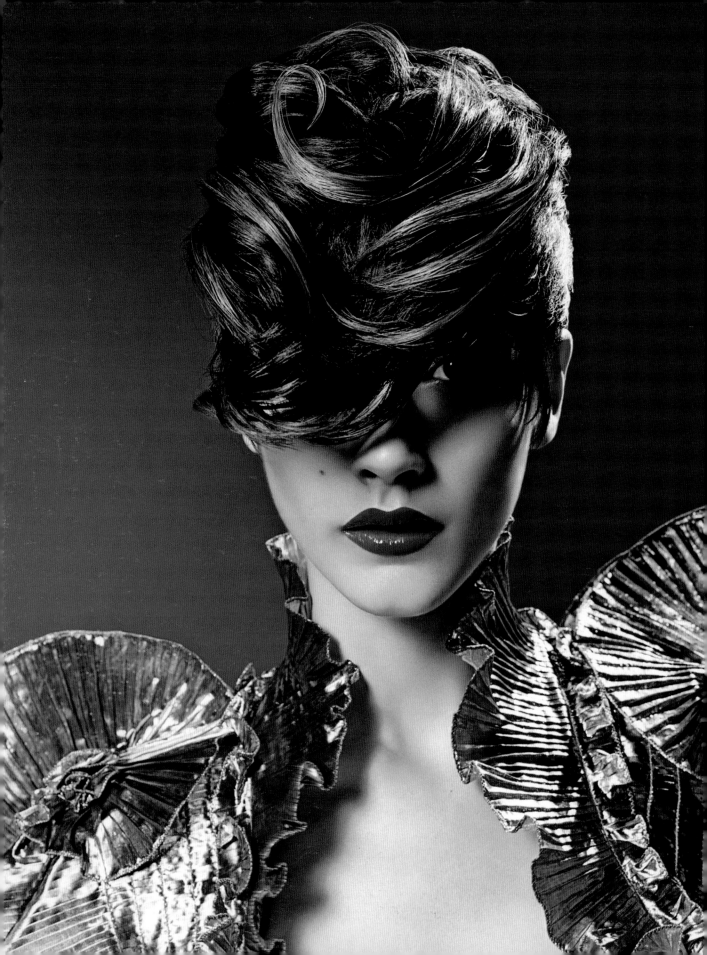

John Nollet

Artistic Designer
L'Oréal Professionel

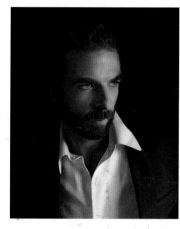

Filled with boldface names from Monica Bellucci (and Vincent Cassel) to Vanessa Paradis (and Johnny Depp), Catherine Deneuve to Audrey Tautou, his little black book is the envy of even the greatest casting directors. But this experimental artist, who has moved into directing with his film Process, *is also a master of color.*

"I never considered any other career than styling women's hair."

Things fell into place very early on for me—thanks to the women in my family who humored me upon returning from the hairdresser's: They gave me the idea of a before-and-after, and it was like magic!

I got my first professional styling head for Christmas when I was 8, then a subscription to *Coiffures de Paris (Paris Hairstyles).* My idols were the Carita sisters and Alexandre, who styled Maria Callas, Elizabeth Taylor, and Grace Kelly.

My parents were excellent listeners—if I wanted to be a juggler, they would have been OK with that. And my grandmother was just as supportive.

When I was 11, I stamped my feet because I wanted to work in a salon, and I have not stopped since. I started stylist's school at 15. I moved from Douai to Valenciennes, where I spent days looking for a job so I could pay for school. I laid siege on all the salons of the city. And then I noticed Maurice Fréalle's: The women who left his salon were undeniably the most beautiful! I offered my services to him during vacation times. I made myself indispensable to him, and he trained me very well. I followed him to Perpignan, and after my first show, which added a credential to my life as a salon stylist, I was lured away by Guy Barber and moved to Montpellier. ▶

A gourmet twist: Swirls of dark chocolate and milk chocolate with long sections swept forward for a bouffant effect.

"Monica Bellucci requests me everywhere: I finally understood that it wasn't to make me happy!"

My next-door neighbor, who was a dancer, changed my life. His friend, the choreographer Dominique Bagouet, was the creator of the Montpelier dance festival. Through them, I discovered contemporary dance, and the company came to have their hair done where I worked. They asked me to create the hairstyles for a play inspired by Lichtenstein and Warhol, and I understood what brought me to this profession. I began working occasionally with the opera as well.

ON THE OTHER SIDE OF THE SCREEN: A FABULOUS DESTINY

The film *Le Retour de Casanova* with Delon, Elsa, and Lucchini, was my first step, as an extra, in the cinema. I worked on the styles of the era and also wigs. I loved it! Then I worked on *Germinal,* spending three months on the set, and it was amazing.

Finally, my sporadic work paid off! I went to Avignon and met Jean-Christophe Spadiccini, who became the star of special effects, former assistant of Jeunet and Caro—and I was hired as the stylist for *La Cité des Enfants Perdus.* I read the screenplay, and they liked my designs, even though I had no experience.

I worked with the best head operators, decorators, producers, and Jean-Marc Tostivain. I went everywhere with them. **At 22, I was the youngest film technician in France!** With the film *L'appartement,* I met Monica Bellucci, Vincent Cassel (who were still unknown at the time), Sandrine Kiberlain, and Romane Bohringer all on the same day. The relationships built at that time are still intact.

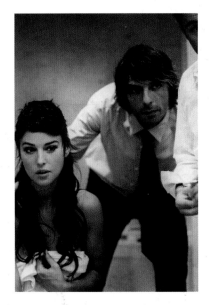

Monica, who has worked with all the stylists in the world as a model, requests me everywhere, telling me she has never found a better stylist. After about 200 times, I finally understood that it wasn't to make me happy. The movie *Ridicule* was a true challenge, with the masked ball and period characters. I proposed to Leconte we use steel wool for the wigs and I produced 200, all while styling the real hair of the admirable Fanny Ardant. She also wore one of my creations the day of the ball. ▶

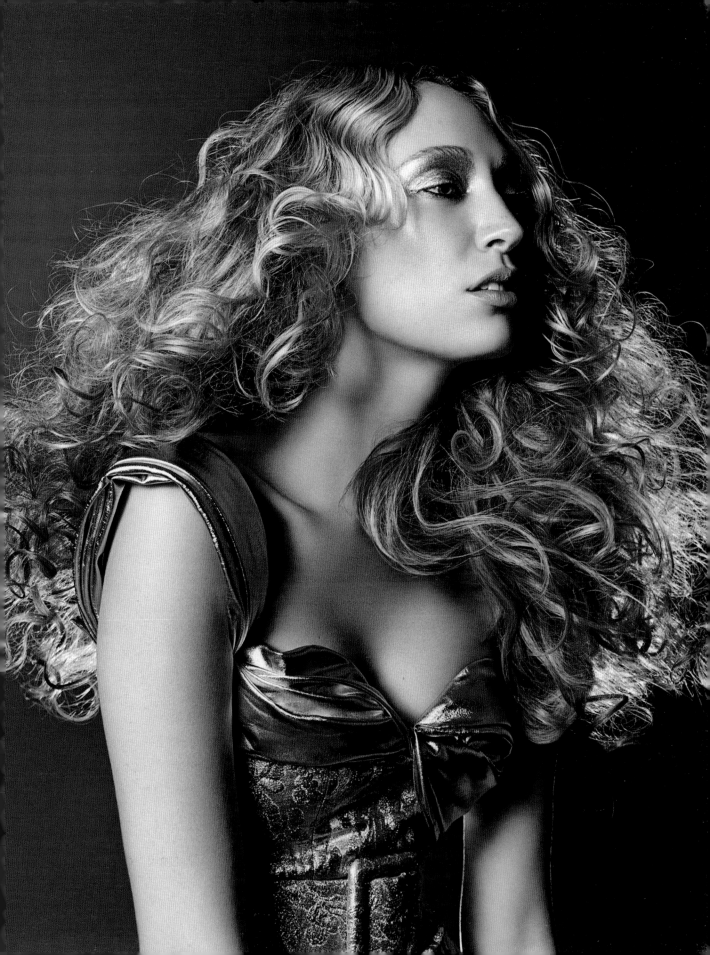

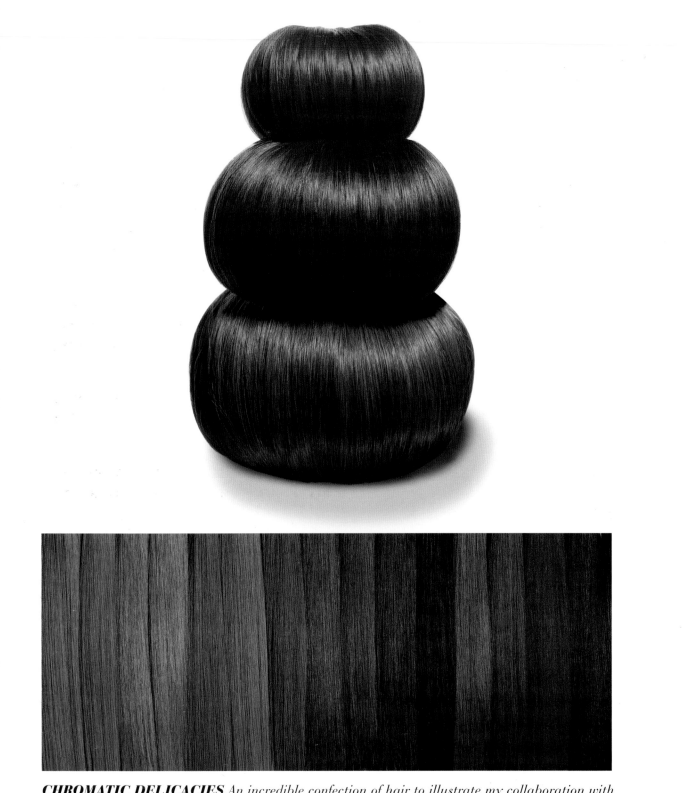

CHROMATIC DELICACIES *An incredible confection of hair to illustrate my collaboration with L'Oréal. In the span of 15 years, I learned amazing techniques and I came away with absolutely everything. Catherine Guillery won me over at a beautiful artistic meeting that launched me into the company, and little by little I did all their images. I became International Creative Director for L'Oréal in 2005.*

"Every woman has the right to be treated like a princess."

I worked on the set of *Une Chance Sur Deux* with Belmondo and Delon and met Vanessa Paradis, and then moved on to *La Fille Sur Le Pont.* It was at that point that Huppert called me for *Rien Ne Va Plus* by Chabrol. Then *Dancer in the Dark* with Deneuve and Björk, by Lars von Trier. On the film *8 Femmes* by François Ozon, I styled three actresses: Catherine Deneuve, Virginie Ledoyen, and Emmanuelle Béart.

Stylists can be crucial to constructing a character. When Jean-Pierre Jeunet let me read his screenplay for *Amélie,* I immediately saw Amélie Poulain in my head. I created the bob hairstyle that Audrey Tautou wore to mark Amélie's style, and now it is impossible to think of her with a ponytail, as Jeunet had imagined. She spends too much time on others to worry about her own appearance!

I moved along to *Astérix, Mission Cléopâtre* and had the opportunity to meet Juliette Binoche, Marion Cottillard, Uma Thurman, Maggie Cheung, Diane Kruger, and Emmanuelle Béart, who called me for Cannes, the Oscars, the Césars.

For *Pirates of the Caribbean,* Johnny Depp asked me to imagine him in the character, and I prepared dreadlocks and decorated them with seashells. I also designed charms and baubles for him, and my creation was interpreted in the film.

All of these experiences change your life, and these are the people who help you to evolve.

I am working on *Mesrine* at the moment, styling a man with a thousand faces. I have created between eight and eleven different heads. I made them in real time, and Vincent Cassel tried them for the filming the next day. I styled Monica Bellucci as a blonde for *Le Deuxième Souffle,* the next film by Corneau, and I have done all of Vanessa Paradis's hairstyles for her album launches.

I opened a salon on Rue Montorgueil with service as precise and attentive as what's offered to stars.

It is an intimate space, where women do not come across each other, where we wash their hair lying down. The fees are not low, but we don't have extra surcharges.

When, at a salon, you are asked the question "Are we washing today?" that usually indicates a surcharge. But not with us!

I also set up shop in the Hotel Costes, and at Cheval Blanc in Courchevel where, as a bonus, we offer hair room service—we bring the salon to the client.

▶

"Your hair is your identity."

My experience has been, when you are very sensitive (which is essential for a stylist), you feel the woman's anxiety and you can anticipate it and diminish it. But women are reassured by the fact that all these famous people have trusted me, and they become more relaxed and ready to participate.

I have never had any pleasure in cutting the hair of a woman who did not want it cut. If she wants to feel long hair down her back, I'm not about to reveal her nape.

MY JOB IS TO FIND THE PERFECT VOLUME. There are hundreds of fashion accessories; you can have the most beautiful dresses and the most spectacular shoes, but the only accessory that you keep when you remove all the others is your hair. It's your identity.

Your haircut is part high fashion and part architecture.

My work is much more than a casual job. It's not a matter of, "If you do poorly at school, you'll be a stylist!"

Designers and chefs, who were simply suppliers a century ago, are stars today, and I am proud of the fact that I am a luxury artisan. The Biennial in Venice, where I presented the performance *La Coupe à Lélastik,* showed how borders have no meaning—and I continued this approach in making *Process,* a film about creation and expression. The film is nine minutes long and is meant to be watched in the dark. It features six scenes which form a sequence from birth to the hatching of a hairstyle. There are also six one-minute "making of" scenes, plus a fifteen minute "making of" by Bilitis Poirier, who is also my artistic collaborator.

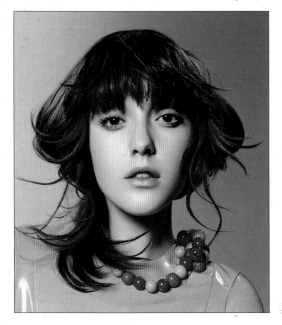

CHOCOLATE CHERRY (at left) or KIWI FLAVOR (at right): the vivid variations that reinvent chestnut by introducing a bit of red and divide blonde into slices to make it stand out and give it spirit.

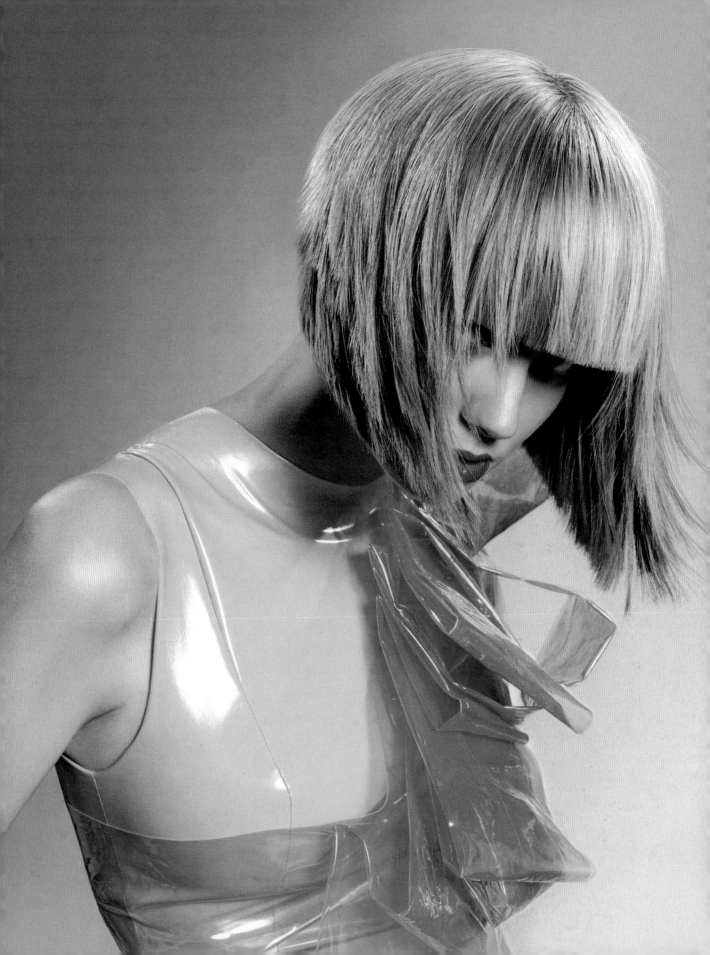

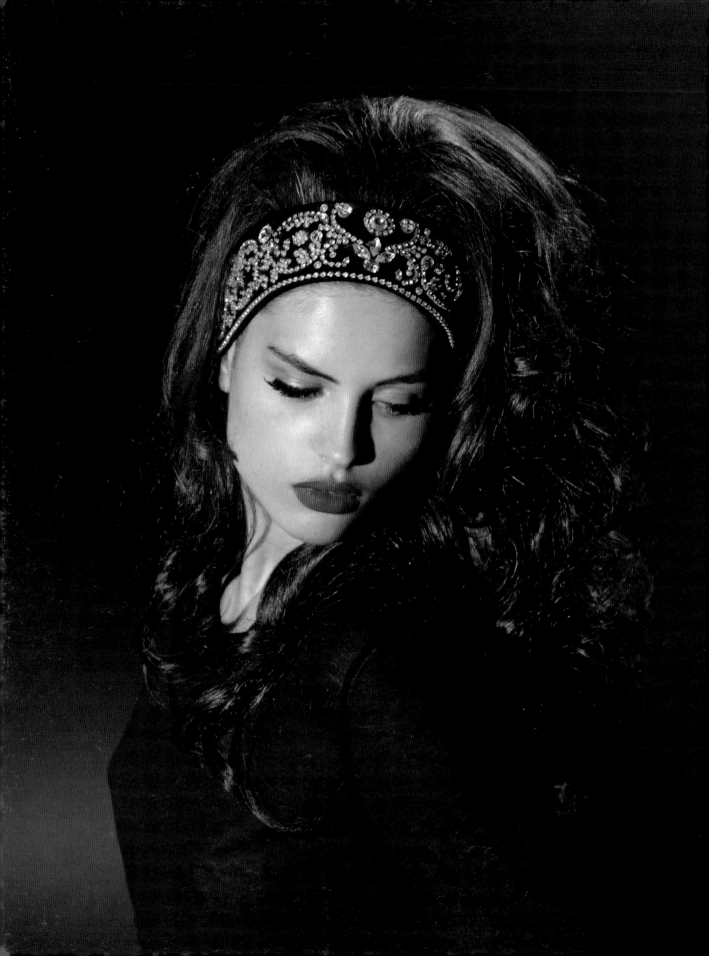

Alexandre Zouari

Hair Designer

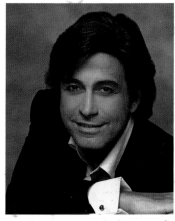

He definitively changed the history of styling by developing his blowdry technique, but the entire career of Alexandre Zouari made him an extraordinary person. He celebrated twenty years in his Paris Maison where actresses, business women, heads of state, and royalty rush in and out. But he still refuses to recognize his own royalty.

> "A **woman** can go without makeup as long as her hair is clean and **beautifully** styled. She can go **anywhere**. The **opposite** is not true!"

THIS CAREER IS ABOUT POWERFUL EMOTIONS AND IMPORTANT MEETINGS, LIKE WITH HER ROYAL HIGHNESS QUEEN RANIA OF JORDAN, who came and asked me to transform her. At 9:30 in the morning, she was a brunette with long straight hair. I called my colorists for her highlights, and she left three hours later with bangs and a layered cut. You know right away when a woman wants to change, but you have to have confidence, you must not fool yourself—this is an enormous responsibility, especially when faced with such an important person.

I also like to remember Carla Bruni with a chignon—I keep that as a dream image, a perfect session. I was lucky, of course, but I also helped it along by working hard. This was an era when women came to have their hair done sometimes three times a day—once for lunch, once for a cocktail party, once for a dinner date—I had up to forty clients a day!

I WORKED WITH THE BIG MAGAZINES AND THE MOST FAMOUS PHOTOGRAPHERS ON A VOLUNTEER BASIS JUST SO I COULD MEET THEM—YOU MUST HAVE PASSION AND BE WILLING TO FIGHT.

▶

I created my collection of jewelry to enhance the most sumptuous manes and put my own twist on the famous saying: Diamonds are your hair's best friend!

"Dare to be bold! But if a woman wants to change everything, you have to trust her … and yourself!"

Helmut Newton and Cecil Beaton (who photographed me, it's still unbelievable), Richard Avedon, Guy Bourdin—I spent entire nights at their photo shoots.

I was brought to this career by love. And I still see it as art. I am never accessible to a large audience, thanks to an elite and very international clientele, which has allowed me to work with all types of hair on all types of women—African, Asian, and American, not simply European. Asian hair is not as soft as European hair, but it is simply marvelous. African hair is very fragile—you need to really take care of it, and most importantly you must not straighten it forcefully. It has texture and beautiful quality, but you have to know how to work with it. African women have beautiful hair, and I love to give them goddess hairstyles.

MY OBSESSION: TO BEAUTIFULLY WORK HAIR. When you run your fingers through a woman's hair, it's magnificent, it's unadorned, it's pure beauty. That's what inspired me to create my jewelry collection. **Today, being a true stylist is not about bending over backward to cut hair.** I have fifty collaborators who all began as assistants: I am very tough in training because being a stylist is not about being content to cut hair and do blowouts. My assistants are always surprised, but there are few people who really know how to style hair these days. Hair is very complicated: Styling is an art, but it's ephemeral. **I prefer to speak of my role as that of revealer—**and more than just in terms of before and after. It's another world, another state of being. A woman can pay no attention to her cut—keeping it natural is fine as long as it's clean—and in this case, she is adapted rather than transformed.

I ALSO DREAM OF PERFUMES. Since time began, women have bathed their hair in perfume essences. My grandmother did it. If you followed a woman's footsteps, she only had to toss her hair, and you'd be able to recognize her fragrance.

SHORT STYLES Women who come in to get their hair cut regularly, who are "crazy for short cuts" are mainly professional women, government workers, journalists, business women. They want to be able to simply wash and brush their hair and have it fall into place on its own. With a good cut and healthy, soft hair, you don't need to blowdry.

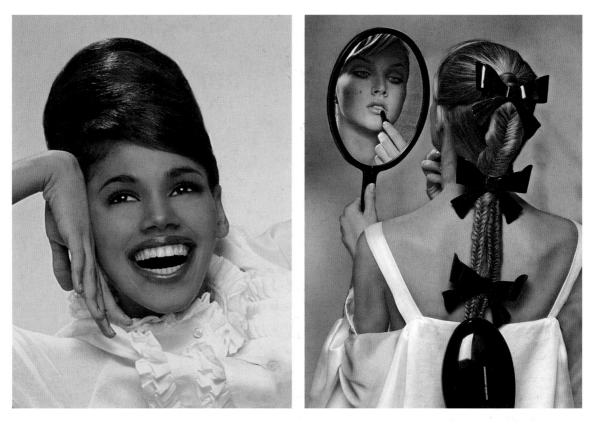

AN UPDATED AUDREY HEPBURN I love this Breakfast at Tiffany's *type of glamour.*
*THE SIRENS OF DESIRE A spectacular sophisticated effect—a summery braid reminiscent of
the stem of an ocean liner . . .*

But before you cut, you must know where you're going—once it's cut, it's too late. You cannot glue it back on. A designer who does not like his dress can go back and change things. With hair, it's not simply a matter of adding fabric—you have to wait two months before it grows back, or have extensions added. **Extensions are such a marvelous resource!** The only disadvantage is, once you're used to seeing yourself with this thick, luxurious mane, you can't go back—when they're removed, you feel like you have no hair!

LONG STYLES Longer hair must be impeccable—clean, shiny, beautifully colored. Long hair is for women who have a bit more time for themselves. We see women come in with ruined hair, dried out by blowdrying. You have to treat it with care, pay attention to it. Creating a perfect, natural look sometimes requires a lot of work!

EXPECTATIONS HAVE CHANGED, AND NOW EVEN MEN WANT TO HAVE THEIR OWN LOOK.

▶

"I recall the blessed era when a woman had her hair done three times a day: for lunch, cocktails, and dinner . . ."

If you want a great sporty cut, proper nourishment is important for hair. You need to eat healthily because your hair, your skin, and your nails are all affected by too much sauces and fats. If you eat poorly, it will be immediately obvious in your skin and hair.

MOST COMMON MISTAKES Changing your hair color every five minutes, having harsh relaxing treatments done, buying a product that is inappropriate for your hair type. The golden rule: Don't go just anywhere for complicated and delicate hair procedures. With regard to the environment and pollution, women are well-informed, but for a haircut they don't know a thing. You must think carefully before launching into something or you may pay dearly.

I'VE STYLED 3,500 BRIDES IN MY LIFETIME—and I'm still able to give them their own original look. The "big day" is back in full force, and every woman has her own vision: It's still magical.

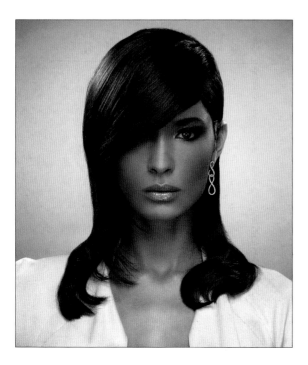

But even the most unbelievable of hairstyles can only last one day while the dress you can keep for a lifetime. The greatest wedding hairstyles are an important part of the history of Maison, they are a Zouari phenomenon. **The chignon is the quintessential evening style, the dress-up style.** You must know all the foundations, like an architect building a house. If the foundation is well situated, if you make the joints properly, then you have only to sculpt, heighten, and do whatever you please!

PHOTO CREDITS

Hugh Arnold (p. 30) ; Edouard Chauvin (p. 4, 5, 36, 101 ; Gilles de Chabaneix (p. 9) ; Greg Conraux (p. 10, 142, 154, 155) ; François Deconinck (p. 4, 62, 63, 73, 76-77, 156, 157/a) ; Bruno Fabbris (p. 51) ; Frédéric Farré (p. 37, 55, 58, 59 ; Hans Feurer (p. 28) ; Guillaume Girardot (p. 34, 35, 43, 46, 47, 96, 147) ; Emmanuelle Hauguel (p. 18/b) ; Bertrand Jacquot (p. 18/a, 18/d, 153/b, 153/d) ; Hermann Jones (p. 160) ; Jean-François Jonvelle (p. 14, 20, 38) ; Bruno Juminer (p. 103, 104) ; Eddy Kohli (p. 29, 39, 56, 60, 86, 89, 140) ; Frédéric Leveugle (p. 74) ; Sarah Maingot (p. 7) ; Jeff Manzetti (p. 41, 42, 45, 48, 52, 78, 82, 83, 145, 149, 161, 164, 165, 166, 167) ; Michel Momy (p. 18/c, 109) ; Marc Montezin (p. 33) ; Pascal Moraiz (p. 85) ; Marc Neuhoff (p. 112, 113/a, 113/b) ; Marc Philbert (p. 157/c) ; Lars Pillman (p. 40) ; Bruno Poinsard (p. 44) ; André Rau (p. 79, 158, 159, 162, 163) ; Bruno Sabastia (p. 143) ; Pierre Sabatier (p. 139) ; Antigone Schilling (p. 25, 27) ; Lothar Schmid (p. 146) ; Massimo Soli (p. 153/a, 153/c) ; Jens Stuart (p. 81) ; Cees Van Gelderen (p. 157/b) ; Patrick Wilen (p. 110) ; Kenneth Willardt (p. 150-151) ; Tobias Zarius (p. 84) ; DR L'Oréal Professionnel (p. 21, 23, 65-71, 93-99, 115-137, 169-188).

HAIR MODEL CREDITS

Céline (p. 161); Christelle (p. 164); **City** Shirley (p. 63, 156); **Contrebande** Phillis (p. 18/a); **Elite** Gaelle Brunet (p. 40, 43, 44); **Delphine Peigne** (p. 158-159); **Ford** Pauline Malingrey (p. 55), Quinn Cooper (p. 81); **Idole** Elodie (p. 142, 143, 145); **IMG** Elena K (p. 18/b); Anastasia Yarubenka (p. 85); Jolijn (p. 78); **Karin** Hélène Dime (p. 18/d); Jessica Lemarie (p. 96); Asia Krol (p. 166); Laurence (p. 167) Louise Deren (p. 79); **Lucie Robinson** Marie Bartosova (p. 41, 42, 45); **Mademoiselle** Julia A. (p. 59); Marie-Martine (p. 162-163); **Marilyn** Maria Gregersen (p. 48, 52, 83); Gili Saar (p. 84); Maryline Fachon (p. 165); **Metropolitan** Elena Soldatova (p. 39, 89); Sandrine Vargas (p. 112, 113/a); Elena Safonova (p. 153/a, 153/c); Mickaela (p. 160); Marta (p. 146, 147, 149); **Next** Anne Flore (p. 7/c); Emma Heming (p. 20); Daniela Kanter (p. 150-151) **Viva-Paris** Caroline de Maigret (p. 76-77/b); Milasgros (p. 18/c); Steffie Davids (p. 154-155); **Women** Charlotte Flossaut (p. 21); **Women Management** Connie Houston (p. 104); **DR L'Oréal Professionnel** (p. 21, 23, 65–71, 93–99, 115–137, 169–191)

Original title: Hair
Copyright 2006 by Editions Marie Claire-Societe d'Information et de Creations (SIC)
www.marieclairebooks.com

General Director, Marie Claire Album SA: Arnaud de Contades
President, Marie Claire Album SA: Evelyne Prousost-Berry

Production Editor: Thierry Lamarre
Author and Editorial Director: Josette Milgram
English Translation: Josette Milgram
Creative Director and Layout Designer: Valerie Paturel
Copy Editor: Julie Bavant
Editorial Assistant: Adeline Lobut
Art Department: Domitille Peyron, Sylvie Creusy, Isabelle Teboul

Library of Congress Cataloging-in-Publication Data
Marie Claire : hair / from the editors of Marie Claire magazine.
    p. cm.
 ISBN 978-1-58816-689-0
 1. Hair—Care and hygiene. I. Marie Claire magazine.
 RL91.M273 2008
 646.7'24—dc22

                        2008016378

10   9   8   7   6   5   4   3   2   1

Published by Hearst Books
A division of Sterling Publishing Co., Inc.
387 Park Avenue South, New York, NY 10016

Marie Claire is a trademark of, and is used under license from, Marie Claire Album.
Hearst Books is a trademark owned by Hearst Communications, Inc.

www.marieclaire.com

Distributed in Canada by Sterling Publishing
c/o Canadian Manda Group, 165 Dufferin Street
Toronto, Ontario, Canada M6K 3H6

For information about custom editions, special sales, premium and corporate purchases, please contact Sterling Special Sales Department at 800-805-5489 or specialsales@sterlingpublishing.com.

Manufactured in China

Sterling ISBN 978-1-58816-689-0